Clozapine Handbook

First edition

To my three beautiful girls, Claire, Sophie and Chloe — SB
To Scarlett, George and Roxie — DT

The authors have made every effort to ensure the accuracy of drug dosage and other information contained in this book. However, this does not diminish the requirement to exercise clinical judgement, and the authors and publisher cannot accept responsibility for the use of the information in clinical practice. Any products referred to by the authors should only be used as recommended in the manufacturers' data sheets.

Clozapine Handbook

First edition

Stephen Bleakley and David Taylor

LRC Lloyd-Reinhold Communications

Lloyd-Reinhold Communications LLP, Dorsington, Warwickshire, UK

British Library Cataloguing-in-Publication Data
A catalogue record is available for this book

ISBN-13 978-0-9569156-1-0

Printed in the UK by Page Bros Ltd, Mile Cross Lane, Norwich, Norfolk, NR6 6SA

Contents

Foreword

I am very pleased to provide a preface to this valuable and timely handbook. Stephen Bleakley and David Taylor have done a service to the field in providing a thorough and well-researched summary of current knowledge regarding clozapine. Given clozapine's continuing unique role in our therapeutic armamentarium, it is valuable to have such a text as a ready resource. It is particularly important since in many countries around the world (and especially the United States), clozapine remains strikingly underutilised and treatment is often inordinately delayed. While the reasons for such limitations in its use are varied, one factor is clearly prescriber concern about the risk and management of a variety of adverse effects. This handbook provides a comprehensive and highly clinically relevant discussion of potential side-effects, as well as the use of clozapine in special populations and complex patient groups. The availability of such information in a user-friendly, single source can help to make such information more readily available to those prescribing or contemplating the prescription of clozapine.

The book will also, no doubt, prove useful to a range of healthcare professionals and even those patients and families who wish to have a rich and scientific source of information on a treatment which might play a very important role in their lives.

As the authors suggest, 'with close monitoring for adverse effects and a slow, cautious titration, there are few absolute contraindications to initiating clozapine. In most (perhaps all) people with treatment-resistant schizophrenia, clozapine offers the best hope of recovery'.

The availability of this handbook should help to facilitate the appropriate use of this unique medication and have a positive and far-reaching impact on the lives of many patients and families around the world.

John Kane M.D.
New York
August, 2013

Introduction

It is astonishing that one of the world's most uniquely effective, yet complex and difficult-to-use drugs for a serious and enduring condition has not had its own book. All the combined data, knowledge and experience dispersed should be shared for the common good. Thus, I congratulate Stephen Bleakley and David Taylor for not only recognising this omission, but also actually doing something about it, and in style too.

This is the first time that all the important and relevant information on clozapine has been assembled in a single, readable and accessible volume, complete with useful summaries. I know that the authors have made a particular effort to include all relevant data up to April 2013, using MedLine, Embase, Psych Info and cross-referenced via Google Scholar, as well as using their own extensive clinical expertise and experience. Thus, all recommendations are reliably evidence-based.

I am particularly pleased to see a dedicated section on post-mortem redistribution (PMR), with the studies summarised concisely. I have had several 'run-ins' with pathologists convinced that (apparent) toxic levels 24 hours after death are conclusive of deliberate overdose and hence suicide. One even failed to shift from this view despite a clearly normal level taken in an acute hospital 30 minutes before the person's tragic death. I fear that some 'suicides' attributed to clozapine overdose may actually be the result of PMR, and so this chapter (with expert contributions from the people's clinical scientist Bob Flanagan) can only help to ensure that accidental death is not classed as suicide.

Clozapine needed its own text book and now it has one, and most enlightening it is too. Thanks guys. You've done a great service to professionals, service users and carers across the world.

Professor Stephen Bazire
Norfolk
August, 2013

Acknowledgements

The authors would like to thank the following people for their enthusiastic support and words of wisdom: Maria O'Hagan, Rebecca Henry, Binkie Mais, Stephen Bazire, Steve Chung, Delia Bishara, Robert Flanagan, Stella Scott, Jo Fabling, Richard Holt, the many members of the College of Mental Health Pharmacy (CMHP) for their continued encouragement, and their families for their boundless patience and understanding.

They also wish to extend their special thanks to Dr Fiona Gaughran of the UK National Psychosis Unit for her help and advice.

1. History and evidence for clozapine's efficacy

The story of how clozapine came to be the widely used drug that it is today is unusual and remarkable. It tells of the triumph of observation over dogma and makes one wonder how many other 'clozapines' have been rejected at an early stage on the basis of perceived scientific laws. The history of clozapine is also the tale of dogged persistence shown by a few caring clinicians who sensed that clozapine was in some way special and refused to let it be killed off.

Early years

The starting point for this story is the near accidental use of chlorpromazine in patients with psychosis in France in the early 1950s. Chlorpromazine is, of course, a phenothiazine compound: two benzene rings surround a six-membered ring containing a sulphur and nitrogen atom, the nitrogen atom bonded to an external carbon chain of various lengths. As word spread of the efficacy of chlorpromazine, several manufacturers began synthesising and testing similar compounds. One of these was imipramine, a tricyclic (as, in the broadest sense, is chlorpromazine) and close chemical congener. The key difference in their structures was that imipramine had a seven-membered nitrogen-containing central ring structure.

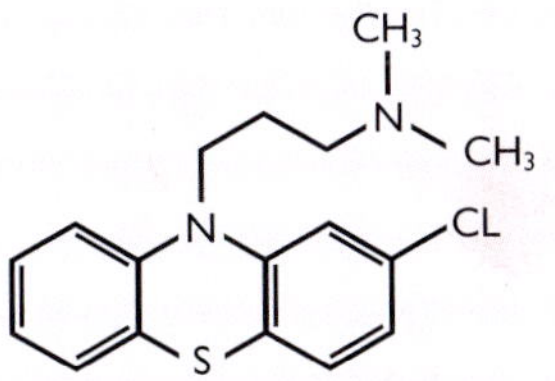

Chlorpromazine

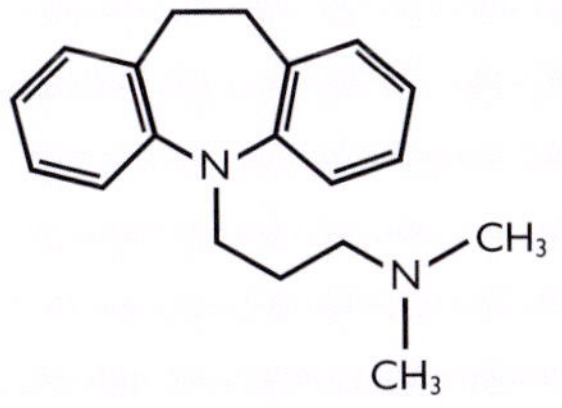

Imipramine

Imipramine was tested in psychosis but found to have no effect. In those with depression it was shown to be thymoleptic — it improved mood, being an antidepressant in most and pro-manic in a few. It was decided that the reason for the different actions of the drugs was the three dimensional conformation of their ring structures. Chlorpromazine's outer rings sat at an angle to the central ring in a butterfly shape, whereas the three rings of the imipramine structure formed more of a 'boat' structure with smaller angles between ring planes. From this observation, manufacturers began synthesising boat-shaped dibenzazepine structures (tricyclics) as antidepressants, and three-ringed butterfly structures (phenothiazines, thioxanthines) as antipsychotics.

Clozapine, was one of a number of compounds synthesised by Wander Laboratories in the late 1950s. Chemically, it is a dibenzodiazepine, its ring structure differing from imipramine by the insertion of a nitrogen atom on one side of the 'carbon bridge' of the seven-membered central ring. Its structural conformation suggested it would have antidepressant properties. In fact, a similar compound produced at this time (dibenzepin) was found to be an antidepressant and is still in use.

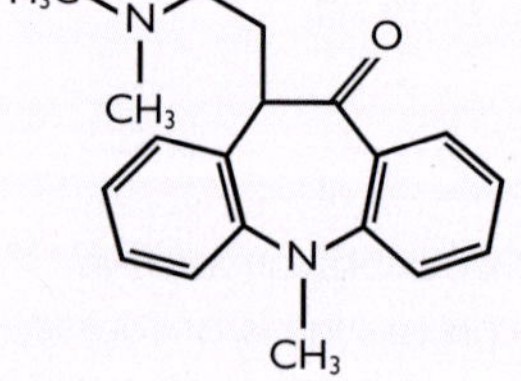

Dibenzepin

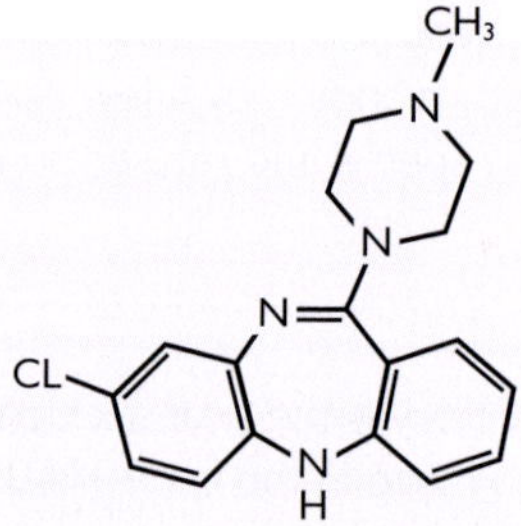

Clozapine

Clozapine was not active in animal screening tests for antipsychotic activity, but its effects in humans were reported to be profoundly antipsychotic and, uniquely, to occur in the absence of extrapyramidal side-effects (EPSE). The Wander company were apparently reluctant to market clozapine as an antipsychotic because it did not fit the prevailing theories on antipsychotic action – all antipsychotics caused extrapyramidal side-effects and so these effects must be part of the antipsychotic action[1].

Demonstrating efficacy

Open label studies of clozapine's effects in schizophrenia were published in German in the mid to late 1960s[2] and by the end of 1966, nearly 100 subjects had received clozapine[3]. The original manufacturers, Wander AG, were acquired by Sandoz in 1967 and clinical testing was increased. Sandoz had already marketed thioridazine and had significant presence in Europe. By the end of 1969, patient exposures had risen to 2200 despite mass prejudice against a drug which produced no EPSE[3].

The first double-blind trial of clozapine (or HF 1854 as it was then known), was reported in 1971[4]. In this study of 64 subjects, clozapine was compared with levomepromazine. Subjects were diagnosed with schizophrenia or mania. Clozapine was more effective against psychotic symptoms than levomepromazine and appeared to act more quickly. Both drugs were sedative; adverse effects noted for clozapine were lowered blood pressure, tachycardia, weight gain and constipation. No EPSE were observed.

In the following few years, a series of small (and so, underpowered) studies were reported showing that clozapine was broadly equivalent in efficacy to perphenazine[5,6], haloperidol[7] and chlorpromazine[8], but with some minor advantages for clozapine noted (against negative symptoms and conceptual disorganisation). Studies reported in the later 1970s were often similarly underpowered, but clozapine's superiority over chlorpromazine with respect to speed of onset and magnitude of positive and negative symptom score reduction was nonetheless detected[9-11]. Clozapine did not show any signs of EPSE in any of the studies conducted in the 1970s.

Agranulocytosis

Phenothiazines have long been observed to be capable of inducing agranulocytosis and some psychiatrists had even called for mandatory blood monitoring for these drugs[12,13]. Thus, by the 1970s blood dyscrasia was a well recognised risk of antipsychotic treatment, although something that was seen only rarely.

In 1975, Finnish workers from the National Board of Health and major Finnish universities[14] reported a sudden rise in the reported cases of agranulocytosis: 18 in 1975 compared with 5–12 in previous years. All 18 occurred in patients given clozapine, which had been introduced to Finland in February 1975. Nine patients died and clozapine use was suspended. Limited analysis suggested a rate of agranulocytosis of around one in 100 patients treated and a mean time to onset of 58 days[14]. Re-analysis by the same authors[15] revised the number of cases to 17 (eight deaths) in 3000 patients treated (i.e. about 0.5% of patients). There was no link to dose, geography (although cases were concentrated in South and West Finland), or purity of the product. Yet more re-analysis by Sandoz[16] reduced the number of cases of blood dyscrasia to 16, agranulocytosis to 13 and deaths to eight. No genetic link could be found between the cases in this analysis or in a further epidemiological study[17]. All reviewers of the situation ascribed the cases of agranulocytosis directly to clozapine[15-17] and weekly monitoring of blood counts was ultimately recommended[18].

Registration

The design and conduct of the preliminary studies outlined above predate full appreciation of clozapine's propensity to cause life-threatening agranulocytosis. In addition, of the two major controlled trials used ultimately to support the registration of clozapine in 1990, one[19] was halted halfway through the recruitment phase because the risk of agranulocytosis was thought likely to be the end of clozapine's development. As a consequence, clozapine eventually achieved widespread release on the basis of only two studies and a total of 419 subjects, of whom only 217 had received clozapine. This remarkable regulatory feat serves as testament to the efficacy of clozapine observed in these studies, and the methods and outcomes of the studies are worth examining in some detail.

The first of the two studies published was lead by James Claghorn, a Texas psychiatrist, and was titled 'The risks and benefits of clozapine versus chlorpromazine' and published in a middle-ranking journal, the *Journal of Clinical Psychopharmacology*[19]. The method section described statistical analyses performed but gives no justification (by means of a 'power' calculation) for subject numbers or dates for the study. (Thus, the fact that this was a half-completed study from the 1970s is not revealed.) The study's provenance is however hinted at by the type of patient enrolled – those with 'neurological reactions to two prior antipsychotics who were symptomatic despite treatment' (although resistance to treatment is not mentioned). In total, 151 subjects took part (300 were intended), of whom a fifth had tardive dyskinesia (another sign of the times, perhaps). At a mean dose of around 400mg a day, clozapine was clearly superior to chlorpromazine (at around 800mg a day) in respect to overall symptom change, time to symptom change and improvement in EPSE. The differences between the two drugs were rather small. Nonetheless, this was probably the first study since the discovery of chlorpromazine to show an unequivocal therapeutic advantage for one antipsychotic over another. Clozapine was more effective and better tolerated than chlorpromazine.

The second study is one of the most famous studies in psychiatry – John Kane's 'Clozapine for the treatment-resistant schizophrenic' (also know as Study 30) published in the most cited psychiatric journal, *The Archives of General Psychiatry*[20]. The trial began in 1984. Kane extrapolated from findings of clozapine's superiority in unselected patient groups to posit that clozapine's place in therapy might be in the treatment of more severely ill and treatment-refractory patients. Indeed, given its then well-known risk of agranulocytosis, this might be the only group of patients in whom the risk was worth accepting.

Subjects in this trial had to have shown a failure to respond to three separate antipsychotics over the previous five years. The antipsychotics had to have been given for at least six weeks at a dose greater than the equivalent of 1000mg/day chlorpromazine. Not satisfied that these criteria could irrefutably demonstrate treatment resistance, Kane enrolled all subjects into a prospective period of treatment with high dose haloperidol (mean 61mg/day). Only five of 305 subjects (1.6%) responded to haloperidol and were duly excluded from the trial proper. Of the remainder, 268 patients were ultimately randomised to either clozapine (up to 900mg/day) or chlorpromazine (up to 1800mg/day, with benztropine). Benztropine was given to all chlorpromazine subjects to help blinding — neither drug would be expected to cause EPSE.

Clozapine was significantly superior to chlorpromazine from the end of the first week of the study. By the end of the study, 30% of subjects on clozapine had met response criteria, compared with only 4% of those on chlorpromazine and benztropine. In addition, improvement in symptoms scores in the clozapine group was fairly uniform over the six-week study period, with no sign of any plateau in effect by this time. Clozapine outperformed chlorpromazine on all efficacy measures in all symptom domains, showing a marked effect in improving negative symptoms which had not been seen before with any drug. This superior efficacy was not achieved at the expense of tolerability — nearly 90% of subjects in both groups completed the trial.

Kane's study was followed up a year later by the publication of findings of a longer term analysis of clozapine response[21]. This was an open, observational study of 51 patients with well-defined treatment-resistant schizophrenia. Its origins were in the observation that Kane's subjects were still improving at six weeks and the suggestion that a longer treatment period might lead to an even better outcome. In Meltzer's study, 27.5% of patients met response criteria (>20% drop in BPRS) at six weeks. This was less than half of those who would eventually be classified as responders. A further 17.6% met response criteria between six weeks and three months and another 15.7% between three months and 12 months (61% response rate overall). Mean reductions in Brief Psychiatric Rating Scale (BPRS) score occurred throughout the 12-month study period but the extent of change reduced over time. Quality of life was also significantly improved.

Most of what we have come to understand about the therapeutic effects of clozapine was first revealed in these studies published in the late 1980s:

- Clozapine shows its superiority best in refractory patients
- 30% might be expected to respond by six weeks
- 60% by a year
- Positive and negative symptoms are improved
- Quality of life is improved.

Other studies in that decade demonstrated clozapine's safety and efficacy in tardive dyskinesia[22] and in long-term maintenance[23].

Since then, we have learned little more about the absolute and relative clinical effectiveness of clozapine. Some studies conducted in the 1990s appeared to show that newer atypicals such as risperidone[24] and olanzapine[25] were just as effective as clozapine. However, this was mere prestidigitation: subjects were often treatment-intolerant rather than treatment-refractory, and clozapine dose was often not properly optimised. Well-conducted studies showed clozapine's clear superiority[26,27].

In this century, clozapine's effectiveness in preventing suicidal thoughts and actions has been demonstrated in a large scale clinical trial[28] and in an observational study of a clinical population[29]. Most recently, the vogue for naturalistic clinical effectiveness studies has confirmed clozapine's superiority over other atypical drugs in treating refractory schizophrenia[30–32]. In the CATIE study, clozapine out-performed other atypicals on nearly all measures, including time to withdrawal and change in Positive and Negative Syndrome Scale (PANSS) score[30]. In these refractory subjects, risperidone and quetiapine had no effect at all and olanzapine only a minor effect. Clozapine, on the other hand, showed robust and clinically useful improvements. In the UK CUtLASS study[31], clozapine again gave better outcomes than other atypicals (amisulpride, olanzapine, quetiapine, risperidone) over the year-long study (but failed to show significant advantages in quality of life). Clozapine's association with improvements in quality of life are yet to be substantiated and quantified, but there is clear evidence of widespread patient satisfaction[33].

Clozapine started out as a putative antidepressant and now, at the time of writing, is in its third decade as the acknowledged most effective antipsychotic available. It is still widely used despite its vast array of adverse effects simply because, even to the naked eye, it is clearly more effective than anything else. The search for a non-toxic clozapine continues with no candidate yet in sight.

Summary

- Clozapine was synthesized as a putative antidepressant in the 1950s.
- Its lack of EPSE prevented widespread use as an antipsychotic.
- By the mid-1970s clozapine had been established as an effective antipsychotic.
- Finnish reports of clozapine-related agranulocytosis lead to its withdrawal around the world.
- American research eventually showed that clozapine was uniquely effective in refractory schizophrenia.
- Recent effectiveness studies have confirmed clozapine's superiority over other antipsychotics.
- Clozapine remains the drug of choice in resistant psychosis.

References

1. Hippius H. The history of clozapine. *Psychopharmacology* 1989; **99 Suppl:** S3–S5
2. Hippius H. A historical perspective of clozapine. *J Clin Psychiatry* 1999; **60 Suppl 12:** 22–3
3. Crilly J. The history of clozapine and its emergence in the US market: a review and analysis. *Hist Psychiatry* 2007; **18:** 39–60
4. Angst J, Jaenicke U, Padrutt A, Scharfetter C. Ergebnisse eines Doppelblindversuches von HF 1854 (8-Chlor-11-(4-methyl-1-piperazinyl)-5H-dibenzo (b, e) (1,4) diazepin) im Vergleich zu Levomepromazin. *Pharmacopsychiatry* 1971; **4:** 192–200
5. Rodova A, Svestka J, Nahunek K, Ceskova E. A blind comparison of clozapine and perphenazine in schizophrenics. *Act Nerv Super (Praha)* 1973; **15:** 94–5
6. Van Praag HM, Korf J, Dols LC. Clozapine versus perphenazine: the value of the biochemical mode of action of neuroleptics in predicting their therapeutic activity. *Br J Psychiatry* 1976; **129:** 547–55
7. Gerlach J, Koppelhus P, Helweg E, Monrad A. Clozapine and haloperidol in a single-blind cross-over trial:

therapeutic and biochemical aspects in the treatment of schizophrenia. *Acta Psychiatr Scand* 1974; **50:** 410–24
8. Ekblom B, Haggstrom JE. Clozapine (Leponex) compared with chlorpromazine: a double-blind evaluation of pharmacological and clinical properties. *Curr Ther Res Clin Exp* 1974; **16:** 945–57
9. Chiu E, Burrows G, Stevenson J. Double-blind comparison of clozapine with chlorpromazine in acute schizophrenic illness. *Aust N Z J Psychiatry* 1976; **10:** 343–47
10. Shopsin B, Klein H, Aronson M. Clozapine: double-blind control trial in the treatment of acute schizophrenia [proceedings]. *Psychopharmacol Bull* 1978; **14:** 12–15
11. Shopsin B, Klein H, Aaronsom M, Collora M. Clozapine, chlorpromazine, and placebo in newly hospitalized, acutely schizophrenic patients: a controlled, double-blind comparison. *Arch Gen Psychiatry* 1979; **36:** 657–64
12. Pisciotta AV, Ebbe S, Lennon EJ, Metzger GO, Madison FW. Agranulocytosis following administration of phenothiazine derivatives. *Am J Med* 1958; **25:** 210–23
13. Korst DR. Agranulocytosis caused by phenothiazine derivatives. *J Am Med Assoc* 1959; **170:** 2076–81
14. Idanpaan-Heikkila J, Alhava E, Olkinuora M, Palva I. Letter: Clozapine and agranulocytosis. *Lancet* 1975; **2:** 611
15. Idanpaan-Heikkila J, Alhava E, Olkinuora M, Palva IP. Agranulocytosis during treatment with chlozapine. *Eur J Clin Pharmacol* 1977; **11:** 193–8
16. Amsler HA, Teerenhovi L, Barth E, Harjula K, Vuopio P. Agranulocytosis in patients treated with clozapine. A study of the Finnish epidemic. *Acta Psychiatr Scand* 1977; **56:** 241–8
17. de la CA, Kari C, Nurminen M, Hernberg S. Clozapine-induced agranulocytosis. A genetic and epidemiologic study. *Hum Genet* 1977; **37:** 183–94
18. Anderman B, Griffith RW. Clozapine-induced agranulocytosis: a situation report up to August 1976. *Eur J Clin Pharmacol* 1977; **11:** 199–201
19. Claghorn J, Honigfeld G, Abuzzahab FS, Sr, Wang R, Steinbook R, Tuason V, et al. The risks and benefits of clozapine versus chlorpromazine. *J Clin Psychopharmacol* 1987; **7:** 377–84
20. Kane J, Honigfeld G, Singer J, Meltzer H. Clozapine for the treatment-resistant schizophrenic. A double-blind comparison with chlorpromazine. *Arch Gen Psychiatry* 1988; **45:** 789–96
21. Meltzer HY, Bastani B, Kwon KY, Ramirez LF, Burnett S, Sharpe J. A prospective study of clozapine in treatment-resistant schizophrenic patients. I. Preliminary report. *Psychopharmacology* 1989; **99 Suppl:** S68–S72
22. Lieberman J, Johns C, Cooper T, Pollack S, Kane J. Clozapine pharmacology and tardive dyskinesia. *Psychopharmacology* 1989; **99 Suppl 1:** S54–S59
23. Lindstrom LH. A retrospective study on the long-term efficacy of clozapine in 96 schizophrenic and schizoaffective patients during a 13-year period. *Psychopharmacology (Berl)* 1989; **99 Suppl:** S84–S86
24. Bondolfi G, Dufour H, Patris M, May JP, Billeter U, Eap CB, et al. Risperidone versus clozapine in treatment-resistant chronic schizophrenia: a randomized double-blind study. The Risperidone Study Group. *Am J Psychiatry* 1998; **155:** 499–504
25. Tollefson GD, Birkett MA, Kiesler GM, Wood AJ. Double-blind comparison of olanzapine versus clozapine in schizophrenic patients clinically eligible for treatment with clozapine. *Biol Psychiatry* 2001; **49:** 52–63
26. Conley RR, Tamminga CA, Kelly DL, Richardson CM. Treatment-resistant schizophrenic patients

respond to clozapine after olanzapine non-response. *Biol Psychiatry* 1999; **46:** 73–7
27. Volavka J, Czobor P, Sheitman B, Lindenmayer JP, Citrome L, McEvoy JP, et al. Clozapine, olanzapine, risperidone, and haloperidol in the treatment of patients with chronic schizophrenia and schizoaffective disorder. *Am J Psychiatry* 2002; **159:** 255–62
28. Meltzer HY, Alphs L, Green AI, Altamura AC, Anand R, Bertoldi A. Clozapine treatment for suicidality in schizophrenia: International Suicide Prevention Trial (InterSePT). *Arch Gen Psychiatry* 2003; **60:** 82–91
29. Tiihonen J, Lonnqvist J, Wahlbeck K, Klaukka T, Tanskanen A, Haukka J. 11-year follow-up of mortality in patients with schizophrenia: a population-based cohort study (FIN11 study). *Lancet* 2009; **374(9690):** 620–7
30. McEvoy JP, Lieberman JA, Stroup TS, Davis SM, Meltzer HY, Rosenheck RA et al. Effectiveness of clozapine versus olanzapine, quetiapine, and risperidone in patients with chronic schizophrenia who did not respond to prior atypical antipsychotic treatment. *Am J Psychiatry* 2006; **163:** 600–10
31. Lewis S, Davies L, Jones P, Barnes T, Murray R, Kerwin R, et al. Randomised controlled trials of conventional antipsychotic versus new atypical drugs, and new atypical drugs versus clozapine, in people with schizophrenia responding poorly to, or intolerant of, current drug treatment. *Health Technol Assess* 2006; **10:** 1–182
32. Attard A, Taylor DM. Comparative effectiveness of atypical antipsychotics in schizophrenia: what have real-world trials taught us? *CNS Drugs* 2012; **26:** 491–508
33. Taylor D, Shapland L, Laverick G, Bond J, Munro J. Clozapine — a survey of patient perceptions. *Psychiatr Bull* 2000; 24: 450–52

1.1: Clozapine in bipolar affective disorder

The extent to which clozapine has been examined in bipolar affective disorder (BAD) is considerably less than that for schizophrenia. Nonetheless, there is little doubt that clozapine is effective in refractory mania and is perhaps the treatment of choice in preventing relapse in refractory or difficult-to-treat bipolar disorder.

Numerous case series attest to the usefulness of clozapine in refractory mania (a condition unlikely to be responsive to placebo effects). For example, Mahmood et al[1] described three cases of mania unresponsive to standard treatments that responded to clozapine in doses around 300mg a day. Another four successful cases were reported by Antonacci and Swartz[2]. Doses used were 150mg/day, 400mg/day and 500mg/day (two patients). Time to full response varied from three to 22 days (all showed complete remission), despite each patient having shown sustained symptoms over several weeks before clozapine was initiated. In a more recent case series of 117 patients from the same unit[3], clozapine (mean dose 353mg/day) showed onset of activity after 2–3 days and decreased Clinical Global Impression (CGI) score[4] from 6.0–4.3 (mean scores for group).

Case reports are of course subject to publication bias since the temptation to publish successful outcomes is much greater than the desire even to submit for publication reports of failed treatments. Prospective studies give a better picture of the extent to which clozapine might be useful albeit, when uncontrolled, without ruling out any placebo effects or the possibility of spontaneous remission occurring independently of drug treatment. Two uncontrolled studies have examined clozapine in treatment-refractory mania. In the first[5], 25 patients received clozapine in doses ranging from 250–800mg a day. Overall, 72% were markedly improved on the Young Mania Rating Scale[6]. In the second[7], 22 patients were given clozapine up to 550mg a day and 77% were ultimately classified as responders. These uniform results are in accord with the only comparative study conducted[8]. In this, 15 patients received a mean dose of 166mg clozapine and 12 chlorpromazine at a mean of 310mg/day. Subjects were not resistant to prior treatment and all received lithium. Clozapine was found to be more rapidly effective than chlorpromazine and more effective overall.

Several observations on these reports are worthy of note. The speed at which clozapine reduced symptoms is remarkable given the need for dose titration. In fact, overall doses tended to be lower than those used in schizophrenia. Perhaps the most striking finding, however, is the proportion of patients who were improved by clozapine — particularly where clozapine was being used in refractory mania.

Prophylaxis

Clozapine's effectiveness in mania might suggest a role for the drug as prophylaxis in BAD, something which had been hinted at when it was relaunched in 1990[9, 10].

A few years later[11] data from a prospective naturalistic study confirmed suspicions to some extent. In all, 17 patients were followed-up for an average of 16.1 months and 11 of the 17 (65%) continued on clozapine alone. None of those 11 patients had relapsed or been re-admitted. A second study[12] compared clozapine (n=19) with treatment as usual (n=19, no clozapine) in patients with treatment-resistant illness with a history of mania. Only three clozapine subjects discontinued (16%), compared with nine of those on treatment as usual (47%). Clozapine was superior on every measure including overall proportion responding to treatment over six months (82% vs 57%). Interestingly, clozapine doses averaged 623mg/day in those with schizoaffective disorder and only 234mg/day in subjects with BAD. The authors concluded that their data supported 'an acute and prophylactic mood-stabilising property of clozapine'.

In the most recent assessment of clozapine's mood-stabilising effects an entirely new approach was used. Nielsen et al[13] accessed the Danish National Patient Registry to discover the fate of BAD patients treated with clozapine. In all, 326 subjects were identified from a register of 21,473 with a diagnosis of BAD (i.e. only 1.5% received clozapine). The mean follow-up time was 544 days and the mean dose of clozapine 307mg/day. By comparing the time before starting clozapine with the time on clozapine, the authors were able to show a mean decrease in bed days spent in hospital from 178 to 35. Overall, nearly three quarters of clozapine patients showed reduced bed stays and nearly 40% were not admitted at all while on clozapine.

Clozapine appears to be effective as an anti-manic and mood-stabilising treatment. Given the data reviewed above, clozapine is probably the drug of choice in treatment refractory BAD. Any certainty over the magnitude of clozapine's effects in BAD are unlikely to be resolved. Randomised, controlled trials are needed to confirm the impressions given by less robust studies already conducted. In the absence of a sole manufacturer of patented clozapine, there is no financial incentive to investigate the role of clozapine in BAD. Ideally, non-commercial funding should be made available for better studies of clozapine in BAD. However, grant-awarding bodies may consider that the case is already proven, especially given clozapine's widespread use in BAD in clinical practice.

Summary

- Clozapine seems to be effective in the treatment of mania, especially that refractory to standard treatments.
- Clozapine also appears to show potent mood-stabilising properties in longer-term treatment.
- There are no blinded, placebo-controlled trials of clozapine in any aspect of bipolar disorder — data are derived from case series, open trials and analysis of patient records.

- The use of clozapine in BAD remains 'off-label' in most countries.
- Clozapine is a reasonable treatment option in refractory BAD. Lower doses may be required than in the treatment of schizophrenia.

References

1. Mahmood T, Devlin M, Silverstone T. Clozapine in the management of bipolar and schizoaffective manic episodes resistant to standard treatment. *Aust N Z J Psychiatry* 1997; **31**: 424–6
2. Antonacci DJ, Swartz CM. Clozapine treatment of euphoric mania. *Ann Clin Psychiatry* 1995; **7**: 203–6.
3. Degner D, Bleich S, Muller P, Hajak G, Adler L, Ruther E. Clozapine in the treatment of mania. *J Neuropsychiatry Clin Neurosci* 2000; **12**: 283
4. Guy W. The Clinical Global Impressions Scale. In: Guy W ed. ECDEU Assessment Manual for Psychopharmacology Rev Ed. Rockville , MD: National Institute of Mental Health; 1976:157–69
5. Calabrese JR, Kimmel SE, Woyshville MJ, Rapport DJ, Faust CJ, Thompson PA, et al. Clozapine for treatment-refractory mania. *Am J Psychiatry* 1996; **153**: 759–64
6. Young RC, Biggs JT, Ziegler VE, Meyer DA. A rating scale for mania: reliability, validity and sensitivity. *Br J Psychiatry* 1978; **133**: 429–35
7. Green AI, Tohen M, Patel JK, Banov M, DuRand C, Berman I, et al. Clozapine in the treatment of refractory psychotic mania. *Am J Psychiatry* 2000; **157**: 982–6
8. Barbini B, Scherillo P, Benedetti F, Crespi G, Colombo C, Smeraldi E. Response to clozapine in acute mania is more rapid than that of chlorpromazine. *Int Clin Psychopharmacol* 1997; **12**: 109–12
9. Naber D, Hippius H. The European experience with use of clozapine. *Hosp Community Psychiatry* 1990; **41**: 886–90
10. Calabrese JR, Meltzer HY, Markovitz PJ. Clozapine prophylaxis in rapid cycling bipolar disorder. *J Clin Psychopharmacol* 1991; **11**: 396–7
11. Zarate CA, Jr., Tohen M, Banov MD, Weiss MK, Cole JO. Is clozapine a mood stabilizer? *J Clin Psychiatry* 1995; **56**: 108–12
12. Suppes T, Webb A, Paul B, Carmody T, Kraemer H, Rush AJ. Clinical outcome in a randomized 1-year trial of clozapine versus treatment as usual for patients with treatment-resistant illness and a history of mania. *Am J Psychiatry* 1999; **156**: 1164–69
13. Nielsen J, Kane JM, Correll CU. Real-world effectiveness of clozapine in patients with bipolar disorder: results from a 2-year mirror-image study. *Bipolar Disord* 2012; **14**: 863–9

2. Mechanism of action

The title of this chapter strikes a teasingly confident tone and the reader is to be forgiven for expecting to read how clozapine manages to be so different from other antipsychotics — to be effective when other drugs have failed. Sadly, no one knows which pharmacological properties or combination of properties are responsible for clozapine's unique therapeutic effects. We know a great deal about the receptor activities of clozapine, both in animals and in man, but we do not know which of them is important for its therapeutic activity and we do not know why drugs with a similar chemistry and pharmacology (quetiapine, olanzapine, among others) do not share clozapine's unique effects.

Since the first clinical use of clozapine in the 1960s (*Chapter one*), clinicians and scientists have struggled to understand why clozapine is uniquely effective. Theories on its mode of action have changed markedly over the years, but even now we seem no nearer to the answer: at the time of writing no new version of clozapine (i.e. a drug for refractory schizophrenia with less problematic adverse effects) is in development. This means that we will not see a replacement for clozapine until the 2020s at the earliest, and it may take decades longer than this.

The main reason we have not yet cracked the code of clozapine is that our knowledge of neuronal function in the brain lags some way behind our observations of drug action. When clozapine was first synthesised, dopamine had yet to be discovered. Twenty years later we only had a superficial understanding of receptor subtypes. Only in the 1990s did genetic sequencing allow us to see what we now think is the full picture: for each transmitter, a multitude of genetically unique receptors with precise and specific locations in the brain. As we will see, theories on the action of clozapine have changed as our understanding of brain neurochemistry has developed. However, two assumptions about clozapine's mode of action remain intact after more than 50 years of use:

- The first is that its efficacy is in some way linked to its atypicality; that is, its lack of extrapyramidal side-effects (EPSE) is inextricably associated to its effect in refractory schizophrenia
- The second is that its activity is at least partly dependent on its inhibition of dopaminergic transmission.

In fact, neither of these assumptions has any grounding in scientific observation and one or both assumptions might be completely false. The scientific community's willingness to cling to these assumptions in some way serves as an explanation as to why we still do not understand how clozapine exerts its effects.

Historical perspective

The American psychiatrist Herbert Meltzer is probably the world's leading authority on the mechanism of action of clozapine. Writing in 1989, shortly after studies had shown clozapine's unique efficacy[1,2], Meltzer put forward the theory that clozapine was able to antagonise both D_2 and $5HT_2$ receptors (but was a stronger antagonist at $5HT_2$ receptors), and that this made it unique and accounted for its action[2]. In the same paper, Meltzer also noted clozapine's apparently greater affinity for D_1 receptors compared with D_2 receptors but discounted this as a meaningless experimental anomaly. D_1 antagonist drugs were later shown to have no effect in psychosis[3].

A year later, Harvard psychiatrist Peggy Stephens summarised theories of clozapine action[4]. Stephens drew attention to early human experiments showing low striatal binding of clozapine to striatal D_2 receptors[5] and to reproducible animal studies showing clozapine's ability to block cortico-limbic dopaminergic function (so-called A-10 neurones) to a greater extent then nigrostriatal function (A-9 neurones). This preferential activity for neuronal function in an area of the brain most probably associated with psychotic symptoms was put forward as the key to its unique efficacy and atypicality. In so doing, the two properties were more firmly linked. (Clozapine's preferential action in human brains was also confirmed[6,7].) Stephens also noted that thioridazine (which she described as an 'atypical neuroleptic') shared the neuronal selectivity of clozapine, but she failed to mention that it did not share its efficacy. (Thioridazine is a piperidine phenothiazine once widely used until being withdrawn in the 1990s because of concerns over QT prolongation.)

Thus, by the early 1990s two theories of action had been proposed: 'D_2/$5HT_2$ ratio' and 'corticolimbic dopamine selectivity'. Each was put forward to explain both clozapine's atypicality and its unique efficacy.

In 1994, Herbert Meltzer returned to the mystery of clozapine's action armed with a greatly advanced awareness of dopamine and 5HT receptor sub-types[8].In his review, Meltzer begins with an observation which is potentially of great significance but is today passed over. Clozapine is effective, as we know, in L-dopa-induced psychosis and in refractory schizophrenia. However, as Meltzer noted, clozapine plasma levels need only be of the order of 25mcg/L to treat the former, but need to be above 350mcg/L for the latter. This strongly suggests that different receptor activities are responsible for the two effects and perhaps that action in L-dopa psychosis does not involve dopamine antagonism. Interestingly, Meltzer by this time mainly discusses the D_4 activity of clozapine, the receptor having been cloned a few years earlier.

He was then proposing that clozapine was almost unique in its preference for D_4 over D_2 receptors (unique if we forget about melperone), and that this explained its unparalleled efficacy. Alongside this, Meltzer persisted with his theories on serotonergic function, now extended by the cloning of numerous receptor subtypes ($5HT_{2A}$, $5HT_{2C}$, $5HT_6$, $5HT_7$). In particular, clozapine's antagonism of $5HT_{2A}$ receptors is proposed as a key function in its action. Support for this was given as the antipsychotic action of pure $5HT_{2A}$ antagonists amperozide and MDL 100,907.

Meltzer's paper also mentioned developing observations of clozapine's effects on the brain's glutamatergic systems — clozapine (but not haloperidol) increased extracellular glutamate levels in rat cortex and could block some of the effects of phencyclidine, an NMDA receptor antagonist.

Three more theories of action had thus been proposed:

- D_4/D_2 ratio
- $5HT_{2A}$ antagonism
- Glutamate enhancer.

The first two of these were soon to be demolished completely.

In 1995, Italian workers published a comprehensive review of the pharmacology of clozapine, reiterating and adding to the above theories of action[9]. On the basis that clozapine was a more potent antagonist of D_1 receptors than haloperidol, it was suggested that this might explain clozapine's atypicality and efficacy. Noting that D_1 antagonism was also seen to a similar extent with thioridazine and flupenthixol, the authors concluded that a high D_1:D_2 activity ratio might account for clozapine's effects. Theories also emerging in this paper include $5HT_{2C}$ antagonism (seen with clozapine and its metabolites) and $5HT_{1A}$ partial agonism (an action almost unique to clozapine). Neither theory has yet been discounted, but these actions on their own do not provide antipsychotic activity.

Towards the end of the 1990s, clinical trials demonstrated the clinical inactivity of several putative antipsychotics which had been developed on the basis of clozapine's pharmacology. Fananserin, a $D_4/5HT_{2A}$ antagonist, was shown to have no efficacy in schizophrenia[10]. Also, the development of the $5HT_{2A}$ antagonists amperozide and MDL 100,907 was cancelled after disappointing trial results. (MDL 100,907 [known as vilonanserin] is now used in veterinary medicines as a pig tranquilliser.) We can thus discount these actions as likely explanations for clozapine's activity although a role of $5HT_{2C}$ is still possible because the $5HT_{2C}$ antagonist (SR46349B) shows some activity in schizophrenia[11], and $5HT_{2C}$ genetic alterations may predict response to clozapine[12]. Also in the late 1990s, investigations into D_3 receptor polymorphism and clozapine response produced equivocal results[13, 14]. Later studies suggested clozapine's *in vivo* affinity for D_3 receptors was not sufficient to provoke therapeutic action[15]. There are currently D_3 antagonists in development (e.g. SB-277,011A), but these are treatments for stimulant addiction rather than schizophrenia.

In the early part of the present century, attention moved towards the nature of clozapine's interaction with dopamine receptors. The Toronto group, led by Philip Seeman and Shitij Kapur, proposed that some atypical antipsychotics were bound only loosely to dopamine receptors and quickly came off them (the 'fast-off' or 'hit-and-run' theory)[16]. This property was confined to clozapine and quetiapine, two antipsychotics at opposite ends of the efficacy scale, and so it did not explain clozapine's unique effects. What this theory did do, however, was to support the idea that clozapine acted via D_2 receptors. That is, although traditional binding studies[6, 16] showed low striatal dopamine binding for clozapine (and so questioned the role of dopamine), studies examining the timecourse of D_2 binding show very high binding at peak plasma levels[17].

This 'fast-off' theory of clozapine's actions survives today[18]. There is considerable evidence that clozapine quickly dissociates from dopamine receptors in human brains. However, there is no clear link between this action and its special efficacy. In fact, there are suggestions that dopamine antagonism is not important to clozapine's action: when aripiprazole is added to clozapine treatment, patients remain stable despite the fact that aripiprazole's affinity for D_2 receptors is three orders of magnitude higher than clozapine and that it is a partial agonist. Indeed, adding any antipsychotic to clozapine seems if anything to improve patients' condition, rather than worsen it[19].

Over the past ten years, researchers have for the most part concentrated on the glutamatergic mechanisms of actions of clozapine as a means to explaining its effects. Glutamate is the main excitatory neurotransmitter in the brain and interacts with a variety of highly complex receptors. The most important of these is the NMDA receptor, manipulation of which produces myriad psychotropic effects. Glutamate acts as an agonist at NMDA receptors but only in the presence of co-agonists Zn^{++} and glycine. The action of glutamate and glycine is terminated by re-uptake into the pre-synaptic neurone or uptake into local glial cells.

Several aspects of clozapine's pharmacology suggest a glutamatergic action. For example, glutamate levels are higher in patients receiving clozapine than those on other antipsychotics[20]. Also, while glycine is an effective augmenter of antipsychotic action when added to ongoing non-clozapine antipsychotic treatment, it has no effect when added to clozapine[21]. Finally, clozapine has been shown to inhibit central glycine transporter mechanisms and this provides an explanation for higher glutamate levels seen in those on clozapine[3].

This brings us more or less up to date, save for a few possible mechanisms (M4 agonism; specific EEG changes) which have been proposed rather than studied in any depth. The mystery of clozapine's mechanism of action thus remains. It is still not clear which of clozapine's actions are essential to its action and which are redundant. Its effects on dopamine and glutamate are probably important, but even of this we cannot be certain. The most we can say is that clozapine's action probably results from interaction with a number of neuronal systems (*Table 2.1*).

Table 2.1: Suggested mechanism of action

Mechanism	Status
D_1 antagonism	Unlikely contributor to antipsychotic activity
D_2 antagonism	Probably involved in antipsychotic activity. 'Fast-off' properties and (consequent?) limbic selectivity make clozapine 'atypical' and may contribute to unique therapeutic effects
D_3 antagonism	Unlikely contributor to antipsychotic activity
D_4 antagonism	Does not contribute to antipsychotic activity
5-HT_{2A} antagonism	Unlikely contributor to antipsychotic activity
5-HT_{2C} antagonism	Unlikely contributor to antipsychotic activity
5-HT_{1A} partial agonist	Unlikely contributor to antipsychotic activity
Glutamatergic activity	Probable contributor to unique effects of clozapine. Clozapine known to inhibit glycine transporter
Some combination of above actions with or without actions yet to be discovered	Highly likely that actions on numerous transmitter systems gives rise to clozapine's unique effects

References

1. Meltzer HY. Clinical studies on the mechanism of action of clozapine: the dopamine-serotonin hypothesis of schizophrenia. *Psychopharmacology (Berl)* 1989; **99 Suppl:** S18–S27
2. Kane J Honigfeld G, Singer J, Meltzer H. Clozapine for the treatment-resistant schizophrenic. A double-blind comparison with chlorpromazine. *Arch Gen Psychiatry* 1988; **45**: 789–96
3. Javitt DC, Duncan L, Balla A, Sershen H. Inhibition of system A-mediated glycine transport in cortical synaptosomes by therapeutic concentrations of clozapine: implications for mechanisms of action. *Mol Psychiatry* 2005; **10:** 275–87
4. Stephens P.A. review of clozapine: an antipsychotic for treatment-resistant schizophrenia. *Compr Psychiatry* 1990; **31:** 315–26
5. Farde L, Wiesel FA, Halldin C, Sedvall G. Central D2-dopamine receptor occupancy in schizophrenic patients treated with antipsychotic drugs. *Arch Gen Psychiatry* 1988; **45:** 71–6
6. Pilowsky LS, Mulligan RS, Acton PD, Ell PJ, Costa DC, Kerwin RW. Limbic selectivity of clozapine. *Lancet* 1997; **350:** 490–1
7. Grunder G, Landvogt C, Vernaleken I, Buchholz HG, Ondracek J, Siessmeier T, et al. The striatal and extrastriatal D2/D3 receptor-binding profile of clozapine in patients with schizophrenia. *Neuropsychopharmacology* 2006; **31:** 1027–35
8. Meltzer HY. An overview of the mechanism of action of clozapine. *J Clin Psychiatry* 1994; **55 Suppl B:** 47–52
9. Brunello N, Masotto C, Steardo L, Markstein R, Racagni G. New insights into the biology of schizophrenia through the mechanism of action of clozapine. *Neuropsychopharmacology* 1995; **13:** 177–213

10. Truffinet P, Tamminga CA, Fabre LF, Meltzer HY, Riviere ME, Papillon-Downey C. Placebo-controlled study of the D4/5-HT2A antagonist fananserin in the treatment of schizophrenia. *Am J Psychiatry* 1999; **156:** 419–25

11. Meltzer HY, Arvanitis L, Bauer D, Rein W. Placebo-controlled evaluation of four novel compounds for the treatment of schizophrenia and schizoaffective disorder. *Am J Psychiatry* 2004; **161:** 975–84

12. Mancama D, Arranz MJ, Kerwin RW. Genetic predictors of therapeutic response to clozapine: current status of research. *CNS Drugs* 2002; **16:** 317–24

13. Scharfetter J, Chaudhry HR, Hornik K, Fuchs K, Sieghart W, Kasper S, et al. Dopamine D_3 receptor gene polymorphism and response to clozapine in schizophrenic Pakastani patients. *Eur Neuropsychopharmacol* 1999; **10:** 17–20

14. Malhotra AK, Goldman D, Buchanan RW, Rooney W, Clifton A, Kosmidis MH, et al. The dopamine D_3 receptor (DRD3) Ser9Gly polymorphism and schizophrenia: a haplotype relative risk study and association with clozapine response. *Mol Psychiatry* 1998; **3:** 72–5

15. Gross G, Wicke K, Drescher KU. Dopamine D(3) receptor antagonism-still a therapeutic option for the treatment of schizophrenia. *Naunyn Schmiedebergs Arch Pharmacol* 2013; **386**: 155–66

16. Kapur S, Seeman P. Does fast dissociation from the dopamine D2 receptor explain the action of atypical antipsychotics?: A new hypothesis. *Am J Psychiatry* 2001; **158:** 360–9

17. Takano A, Suhara T, Kusumi I, Takahashi Y, Asai Y, Yasuno F, et al. Time course of dopamine D2 receptor occupancy by clozapine with medium and high plasma concentrations. *Prog Neuropsychopharmacol Biol Psychiatry* 2006; **30:** 75–81

18. Vauquelin G, Bostoen S, Vanderheyden P, Seeman P. Clozapine, atypical antipsychotics, and the benefits of fast-off D2 dopamine receptor antagonism. *Naunyn Schmiedebergs Arch Pharmacol* 2012; **385:** 337–72

19. Taylor D, Smith L, Gee SH, Nielsen J. Augmentation of clozapine with a second antipsychotic. A meta analysis. *Acta Psychiatr Scand* 2012; **125:** 15–24

20. Evins AE, Amico ET, Shih V, Goff DC. Clozapine treatment increases serum glutamate and aspartate compared to conventional neuroleptics. *J Neural Transm* 1997; **104:** 761–6

21. Shim SS, Hammonds MD, Kee BS. Potentiation of the NMDA receptor in the treatment of schizophrenia: focused on the glycine site. *Eur Arch Psychiatry Clin Neurosci* 2008; **258:** 16–27

3. Clozapine augmentation

Clozapine is widely recognised as the most efficacious option for those with treatment-resistant schizophrenia[1,2]. Nethertheless, up to 70% of these patients have a poor or inadequate response to clozapine alone[3] and 'augmenting' with another agent has become commonplace in clinical practice[4]. The evidence base supporting augmentation is limited, often conflicting, and at best shows only a marginally improved response[3,5,6]. Before augmentation is considered, clozapine treatment should be optimised, ensuring adequate dose, duration of treatment and adherence (*Figure 3.1*).

Figure 3.1: Factors to consider before clozapine augmentation

- Poor adherence should be investigated and addressed
- Clozapine monotherapy should be tried for at least 3–6 months to evaluate efficacy
- Clozapine plasma levels of at least 350mcg/L should be achieved
- Additional medication may have pharmacokinetic or pharmacodynamic interactions with clozapine
- Combinations may require additional physical health monitoring
- Efficacy should be assessed using recognised scales
- Always time-limit any trial (e.g. 3–6 months) and discontinue the augmenting agent if response is unsatisfactory

Table 3.1 outlines the pharmacological approaches which have been used to augment clozapine. Although the evidence base is developing, questions remain unanswered and many negative results are reported. Augmenting agents with which there are the most published data are lamotrigine, aripiprazole, risperidone and sulpiride. This does not mean that these are the preferred agents, only that they are the best studied. Augmenting clozapine with any antipsychotic shows a small but significant benefit (effect size -0.239)[6], but data are lacking to confirm which antipsychotic combination confers the most benefit[5,6].

Table 3.1. Pharmacological approaches to clozapine augmentation

Drug/type of studies	Typical daily dose	Total nos in RCTs	Duration	Comments
Antiepiletics				
Lamotrigine Six RCTs and one meta-analysis[7]	100–400mg	195	Up to 24 weeks	Meta-analysis suggests a moderate effect size although several negative RCTs exist[8,9]. When effective benefits in both positive and negative symptoms are demonstrated. Generally well tolerated. Monitor closely for a rash during the initial titration of lamotrigine

Table 3.1. Pharmacological approaches to clozapine augmentation *continued*

Topirimate Four RCTs[10,11,12,13], multiple case series[13]	50–400mg	117	Up to 24 weeks	Two positive[10,11] and two negative RCTs[12,13] associated with weight loss, impaired cognition, visual disturbances, depression and psychosis
Antipsychotics				
Amisulpride One RCT[14], one open label study[16] and case series[18].	400–600mg	72	Up to 8 weeks	Trend to improvement seen but failed to reach significance in one small RCT[14]. Greater improvement seen with amisulpride augmentation than quetiapine-clozapine augmentation[15]. An open label study (n=33) reported the benefit continued to 6 months[16]. Occasionally used for clozapine-induced hypersalivation[17]
Aripiprazole Four RCTs[19,20,21,22], many case series and open-labelled studies	15–30mg	407	Up to 12 months follow-up	Limited evidence for an improvement in symptoms. One RCT demonstrated an improvement in positive symptoms only[19], another reported only improvements in negative symptoms[20]. May be as effective as haloperidol and clozapine in combination but better tolerated[20]. May reduce the metabolic risks associated with clozapine[21]
Haloperidol One RCT[22] and case series[23]	2–4mg	106	Up to 12 months follow-up	Shown to be as effective as clozapine and aripiprazole but less well tolerated[22]
Olanzapine Case reports only[24]	15mg	—	Up to 1 year follow-up	Poorly supported and likely to exacerbate metabolic adverse-effects
Paliperidone Case series[25]	6–12mg	—	8 weeks	A subjective improvement in symptoms was observed
Pimozide Two RCTs[26,27]	2–8mg	85	Up to 12 weeks	Two well conducted RCTs failed to demonstrate any improvement in symptoms. Pimozide is associated with QTc prolongation
Risperidone Five RCTs[6] multiple open studies and case reports[28]	2–6mg	114	Up to 18 weeks	Two negative RCTs[29,30]. A lower risperidone dose and longer duration of trial may improve outcome[28]. Comparable efficacy to ziprasidone and clozapine combination, but with a greater rise in serum prolactin[31]
Sertindole One RCT[32]	16 mg	50	Up to 12 weeks	No benefit over placebo shown and associated with QTc prolongation
Sulpiride Four RCTs and a Cochrane review[33]	200–1000mg	221	Up to 12 weeks	Short-term data favoured sulpiride combination over placebo. Overall effect was modest. Mostly Chinese studies

Table 3.1. Pharmacological approaches to clozapine augmentation *continued*				
Ziprasidone One RCT[31], one open study[34], and case series[35]	80–160mg	12	Up to 6 weeks	Comparable efficacy to risperidone and clozapine combination, but associated with QTc prolongation[31]
		Antidepressants		
Duloxetine One RCT[36]	60mg	33	16 weeks	Some benefit in negative symptoms and general psychopathology shown
Fluoxetine One RCT[37]	20–60mg	33	8 weeks	No significant differences were found between fluoxetine and placebo augmentation. Fluoxetine may increase clozapine plasma levels
Mirtazapine One RCT[38]	30mg	24	8 weeks	Some improvements in negative symptoms reported. Associated with weight gain and sedation which may be exacerbated in combination with clozapine
		Others		
Donepezil One small RCT[39]	10mg	8	18 weeks	A trend to an improvement in positive symptoms was seen but this did not reach significance
Glycine Three RCTs[40,41,42]	30–60mg	61	28 weeks	All three RCTs failed to show any improvements in symptoms. One reported a greater improvement in the clozapine monotherapy group[42]
Ginko Biloba One RCT[43]	120mg	42	12 weeks	A significant improvement in negative symptoms was reported. No effect on positive or overall symptomology
Memantine One RCT[44]	20mg	21	12 weeks	Significant improvements in negative and positive symptoms and cognition demonstrated

Combining ECT with clozapine is discussed in *Chapter 10.7, pp. 179–180*

Summary

- Augmenting clozapine with another agent is commonplace in clinical practice but has limited supporting data.
- Augmenting with lamotrigine, aripiprazole, risperidone and sulpiride has been studied the most.
- Any augmenting strategy requires close monitoring for pharmacokinetic and pharmacodynamic drug interactions.
- Improvements in efficacy and tolerability should be carefully assessed during the augmentation.
- If no improvement is evident after 3–6 months, the augmenting agent should be discontinued.

Further reading

Sommer I, Begemann M, Temmerman A, Leucht S. Pharmacological augmentation strategies for schizophrenia patients with insufficient response to clozapine: A quantitative literature review. *Schizophr Bull* 2012; **38:** 1003–11

Taylor D, Smith L, Gee S, Nielsen J. Augmentation of clozapine with a second antipsychotic – a meta-analysis. *Acta Psychiatrica Scand* 2012; **125:** 15–24

References

1. National Collaborating Centre for Mental Health. Schizophrenia: Core Interventions in the Treatment of Schizophrenia in Adults in Primary and Secondary Care (Updated Edition) (NICE Clinical Guideline CG82). National Institute for Health and Clinical Excellence, 2009
2. Barnes T, the Schizophrenia Consensus Group for the British Association for Psychopharmacology. Evidence-based guidelines for the pharmacological treatment of schizophrenia: recommendations from the British Association for Psychopharmacology. *J Psychopharmacology* 2011; **25:** 567–620
3. Sommer I, Begemann M, Temmerman A, Leucht S. Pharmacological augmentation strategies for schizophrenia patients with insufficient response to clozapine: A quantitative literature review. *Schizophr Bull* 2012; **38:** 1003–11
4. Pai N, Laidlow M, Vella S. Augmentation of clozapine with another pharmacological agent: treatment for refractory schizophrenia in the 'real world'. *Acta Psychiatr Scand* 2012; **126:** 40–6
5. Cipriani A, BosoM, Barbui C. Clozapine combined with different antipsychotic drugs for treatment resistant schizophrenia. Cochrane Database of Systematic Reviews 2009, Issue 3. Art. No.: CD006324. DOI: 10.1002/14651858.CD006324.pub2
6. Taylor D, Smith L, Gee S, Nielsen J. Augmentation of clozapine with a second antipsychotic – a meta-analysis. *Acta Psychiatr Scand* 2012; **125:** 15–24
7. Tiihonen J, Wahlbeck K, Kiviniemi V. The efficacy of lamotrigine in clozapine-resistant schizophrenia: a systematic review and meta-analysis. Schizophrenia Research 2009; 109: 10-14.
8. Vaygoglu S, Yagcioglu A, Yagcgoglu S, Karahan S, Karcg O, Gurel S, et al. Lamotrigine augmentation in patients with schizophrenia who show partial response to clozapine treatment. *Schizophr Res* 2013; **143:** 20714
9. Goff D, Keefe R, Citrome L, Davy K, Krystal J, Large C, et al. Lamotrigine as add-on therapy in schizophrenia: results of 2 placebo-controlled trials. *J Clin Psychopharmacol* 2007; **27:** 582–9
10. Hahn M, Remington G, Bois D, Cohn T. Topiramate augmentation in clozapine-treated patients with schizophrenia: clinical and metabolic effects. *J Clin Psychopharmacol* 2010; **30:** 706–10
11. Afshar H. Topiramate add-on treatment in schizophrenia: a randomised, double-blind, placebo-controlled clinical trial. *J Psychopharmacol* 2009; **23:** 157–62
12. Muscatello M, Bruno A, Pandolfo G, Mico U, Bellinghieri P, Scimeca G, et al. Topirimate augmentation of clozapine in schizophrenia: A double-blind, placebo-controlled study. *J Psychopharmacol* 2011; **25:** 667–74
13. Tiihonen J, Halonen P, Wahlbeck K. Topiramate add-on in treatment-resistant schizophrenia: a randomised, double-blind, placebo-controlled, crossover trial. *J Clin Psychiatry* 2005; **66:** 1012–15
14. Assion H, Reinbold H, Lemanski S, Basilowski M, Juckel G. Amisulpride augmentation in patients with schizophrenia partially responsive or unresponsive to clozapine. A randomized, double-blind,

placebo-controlled trial. *Pharmacopsychiatry* 2008; **41**: 24–8

15. Genc Y, Taner E, Candansayear S. Comparison of clozapine-amisulpride and clozapine-quetiapine combinations for patients with schizophrenia who are partially responsive to clozapine: A single-blind randomized study. *Adv Therapy* 2007; **24**: 1–13
16. Munro J, Matthiasson P, Osborne S, Travis M, Purcell S, Cobb A, et al. Amisulpride augmentation of clozapine: an open non-randomized study in patients with schizophrenia partially responsive to clozapine. *Acta Psychiatr Scand* 2004; **110**: 292–8
17. Kreinin A, Novitski D, Weizman A. Amisulpride treatment of clozapine-induced hypersalivation in schizophrenia patients: A randomized, double-blind, placebo-controlled cross-over study. *Int Clin Psychopharmacol* 2006; **21**: 99–103
18. Agelink M, Kavuk I, Ak I. Clozapine with amisulpride for refractory schizophrenia. *Am J Psychiatry* 2004; **161**: 924–5
19. Muscatello M, Bruno A, Pandolfo G, Micò U, Scimeca G, Di Nardo F, et al. Effect of aripiprazole augmentation of clozapine in schizophrenia: a double-blind, placebo-controlled study. *Schizophr Res* 2011; **127**: 93–9
20. Chang J, Ahn Y, Park H, Lee K, Kim S, Kang U, et al. Aripiprazole augmentation in clozapine-treated patients with refractory schizophrenia: an 8-week, randomized, double-blind, placebo-controlled trial. *J Clin Psychiatry* 2008; **69**: 720–31
21. Fleischhacker W, Heikkinen M, Olié J-P, Landsberg W, Dewaele P, McQuade R, et al. Effects of adjunctive treatment with aripiprazole on body weight and clinical efficacy in schizophrenia patients treated with clozapine: a randomized, double-blind, placebo-controlled trial. *Int J Neuropsychopharmacol* 2010; **13**: 1115–25
22. Barbui C, Accordini S, Nose M, Stroup S, Purgato M, Girlanda F, et al. Aripiprazole versus haloperidol in combination with clozapine for treatment-resistant schizophrenia in routine clinical care: A randomized, controlled trial. *J Clin Psychopharmacol* 2011; **31**: 266–73
23. Kapur S, Roy P, Daskalakis J, Remmington G, Zipursky R. Increased dopamine D2 receptor occupancy and elevated prolactin level associated with addition of haloperidol to clozapine. *Am J Psychiatry* 2001; **158**: 311–14
24. Gupta S, Sonnenberg S, Frank B, Olanzapine augmentation of clozapine. *Ann Clin Psychiatry* 1998; **10**: 113–15
25. Chang T, Hsu W, Huang S, Chiu N, Liao Y. Augmentation of clozapine with paliperidone in treatment-resistant schizophrenia. A case series. *Acta Neuropsychiatr* 2011; **23**: 51–3
26. Gunduz-Bruce H, Oliver S, Gueorguieva R, Forselius-Bielen K, D'Souza D, Zimolo Z, et al. Efficacy of pimozide augmentation for clozapine partial responders with schizophrenia. *Schizophr Res* 2013; **143**: 344–7
27. Friedman J, Lindenmayer J, Alcantara F, Bowler S, Parak M, White L, et al. Pimozide augmentation of clozapine in patients with schizophrenia and schizoaffective disorder unresponsive to clozapine. *Neuropsychopharmacoogy* 2011; **36**: 1289–95
28. Kontaxakis V, Ferentinos P, Havaki-Kontaxake B, Paplos K, Pappa D, Christodoulou G. Risperidone augmentation of clozapine. *Eur Arch Psychiatry Clin Neurosci* 2006; **256**: 350–5
29. Freudenreich O, Henderson D, Walsh J, Culhane M, Goff D. Risperidone augmentation for schizophrenia partially responsive to clozapine: a double-blind, placebo-controlled trial. *Schizophr* Res

2007; **92:** 90–4

30. Honer W, Thornton A, Chen E, Chan R, Wong J, Bergmann A, et al. Clozapine alone versus clozapine and risperidone with refractory schizophrenia. *N Engl J Med* 2006; **354:** 472–82
31. Zink M, Kuwilsky A, Krumm B, Dressing H. Efficacy of ziprasidone versus risperidone as augmentation in patients partially responsive to clozapine: a randomised controlled clinical trial. *J Psychopharmacol* 2009; **23:** 305–14
32. Nielsen J, Emborg C, Gydesen S, Dybbro J, Aagaard J, Haderup K, et al. Augmenting clozapine with sertindole: A double-blind, randonized, placebo-controlled study. *J Clin Psychopharmacol* 2012; **32:** 173–8
33. Wang J, Omori IM, Fenton M, Soares BGO. Sulpiride augmentation for schizophrenia. Cochrane Database of Systematic Reviews 2010, Issue 1. Art. No.: CD008125. DOI: 10.1002/14651858.CD008125.pub2
34. Ziegenbein M, Kroop S, Kuenzel H. Combination of clozapine and ziprasidone in treatment-resistant schizophrenia: an open clinical study. *Clin Neuropharmacol* 2005; **28:** 220–4
35. Kaye N. Ziprasidone augmentation of clozapine in 11 patients. *J Clin Psychiatry* 2003; **64:** 215
36. Mico U, Bruno A, Pandolfo G, Romeo M, Mallamance D, D'Arrigo C, et al. Duloxetine as adjunctive treatment to clozapine in patients with schizophrenia: A randomized, placebo-controlled trial. *Int Clin Psychopharmacol* 2011; **26:** 303–10
37. Buchanan R, Kirkpatrick B, Bryant N, Ball P, Breirer A. Fluoxetine augmentation of clozapine treatment in patients with schizophrenia. *Am J Psychiatry* 1996; **153:** 1625–7
38. Zoccali R, Muscatello M, Cedro C, Neri P, La Torre D, Spina E, et al. The effect of mirtazapine augmentation of clozapine in the treatment of negative symptoms of schizophrenia: a double-blind, placebo-controlled study. *Int Clin Psychopharmacol* 2004; **19:** 71–6
39. Stryer R, Strous R, Bar F, Shaked G, Shiloh R, Rozencwaig S, et al. Donepezil augmentation of clozapine monotherapy in schizophrenia patients: a double-blind cross over study. *Hum Psychopharmacol: Clinical and Experimental* 2004; **19:** 343–6
40. Diaz P, Bhaskara S, Dursun S, Deakin B. Double-blind placebo-controlled, crossover trial of clozapine plus glycine in refractory schizophrenia negative results. *J Clin Psychopharmacol* 2005; **25:** 277–8
41. Evins A, Fitzgerald S, Wine L, Rosselli R, Goff D. Placebo-controlled trial of glycine added to clozapine in schizophrenia. *Am J Psychiatry* 2000; **157:** 826–8
42. Potkin S, Jin Y, Bunney B, Costa J, Gulasekaram M. Effect of clozapine and adjunctive high-dose glycine in treatment-resistant schizophrenia. *Am J Psychiatry* 1999; **156:** 145–7
43. Doruk A, Uzun O, Ozsahin A. A placebo-controlled study of extract of ginkgo biloba added to clozapine in patients with treatment-resistant schizophrenia. *Int Clin Psychopharmacol* 2008; **23:** 223–7
44. De Lucena D, Fernandes S, Berk M, Dodd S, Medeiros D, Pedrini M, et al. Improvement of negative and positive symptoms in treatment-refractory schizophrenia: a double-blind, randomized, placebo-controlled trial with memantine as add-on therapy to clozapine. *J Clin Psychiatry* 2009; **70:** 1416–23

4. Initiation and monitoring parameters

Despite robust evidence to support clozapine as the recommended choice for treatment-resistant schizophrenia, it remains underutilised and treatment is often delayed[1]. The National Institute for Health and Clinical Excellence (NICE, 2009) guidelines state that[2]:

> *Clinicians should offer clozapine to people with schizophrenia whose illness has not responded adequately to treatment despite the sequential use of adequate doses of at least two different antipsychotic drugs.*

An appropriate trial of an antipsychotic is usually considered to be 4–6 weeks[2] at an optimum dose. Thus, after a minimum of eight weeks of poor response (or poor tolerability), clozapine should be initiated. In the authors' clinical experience, this is rarely the case and clozapine is often delayed for years and is erroneously considered as the treatment of last resort. In one large London NHS trust, the average delay in initiating clozapine was four years[3], while literature from New Zealand reports a delay of over nine years from first contact with services[4]. Prescribing rates of clozapine also appear to vary across similar services. A study of 45 mental health NHS trusts in England reported a fivefold variation in clozapine prescribing, and only 30% of those eligible for clozapine were actually receiving it[5]. Why clozapine treatment is so delayed is unclear, but may be related to unfamiliarity, concern over the adverse effects and the routine blood test requirements, or lack of active marketing[6]. Clinicians' concerns about using clozapine do not seem to be mirrored by service users. In a UK-wide survey of patient perceptions on clozapine, of 570 responders, 89% claimed to prefer to stay on clozapine rather than change to another drug. Although 24% of the clozapine users mentioned that they did not like the blood tests, most (87%) felt that the advantages of clozapine outweighed the disadvantages[7].

With close monitoring for adverse effects and a slow, cautious titration, there are few absolute contraindications to initiating clozapine. In most (perhaps all) people with treatment-resistant schizophrenia, clozapine offers the best hope of recovery.

Initiating clozapine

Before starting clozapine, patients should undergo a thorough physical health review and any previous health complaints should be investigated. Consideration should be given to potential drug interactions with any prescribed or purchased medication (including herbal products), smoking status of the person (particularly if they are intending to stop smoking), caffeine intake and previous tolerability to other antipsychotics. *Table 4.1* outlines the recommended baseline monitoring parameters ('work-up') before starting clozapine.

Table 4.1: Baseline monitoring parameters before starting clozapine[8,9]
Monitoring parameters
Blood pressure (sitting and standing)
Pulse
Temperature
Respiratory rate monitoring
Urea and electrolytes (including eGFR)
Full blood count (WBCs, neutrophils, eosinophils)
ECG
Blood lipids, fasting sample (cholesterol and triglycerides)
Weight (including BMI, and abdominal circumference)
Plasma glucose (fasting sample ideally)
Liver function tests (ALT, AST, bilirubin, albumin, prothrombin), fasting sample ideally
Troponin T or I
C-reactive protein
EEG (under 16s only)
Investigate potential problems with prescribed, bought or herbal medication, illicit drugs and alcohol
Record current smoking status, caffeine intake, lifestyle and diet
Investigate for any previous history of blood disorders, seizures, DVTs, PEs, cardiac, bowel or bladder dysfunction, glaucoma, OCD and liver or renal impairment

ALT = *alanine aminotransferase*; AST = *aspartate aminotransferase*; BMI = body mass index;
ECG = *electrocardiogram*; EEG = *electroencephalogram*; eGFR = *estimated glomerular filtration rate*;
DVT = *deep vein thrombosis*; OCD = *obsessive compulsive disorder*; PE = *pulmonary embolism*

The potential benefits and risks of clozapine therapy along with the importance of adherence should be fully discussed with the patient, family and carers and they should be given adequate time to ask questions or raise concerns. All discussions and decisions should be fully documented and followed-up by appropriate written information. In the UK, US, Canada, Australia, New Zealand, and Ireland the patient, pharmacy and psychiatrist will need to be registered with the appropriate clozapine company before initiating treatment (*Appendix I*).

Many adverse effects of clozapine are predictable, dose-dependent and often related to the speed of titration. Any emerging adverse effect should precipitate a slowing down or freezing of the titration or, if intolerable, a reduction in the clozapine dose to one previously tolerated. *Table 4.2* suggests a cautious dose regimen for initiating clozapine for people who are inpatients. Faster titrations have been used in those who have previously tolerated clozapine. Equally, slower titrations may be appropriate for the elderly, the very young, those who are physically compromised, or for those who have poorly tolerated other antipsychotics. The monitoring parameters listed in *Table 4.2* are suggested as the minimum required and some vulnerable patient groups may require more intensive monitoring. The target doses are taken from clozapine RCTs or the average dose reported to achieve the minimum therapeutic plasma levels[10]. After initial titration, patients should be maintained on the lowest effective clozapine dose.

Table 4.2: Dosing and monitoring regimen for inpatients[8, 9]

Day	Morning dose (mg)	Evening dose (mg)*	Total daily dose (mg)	Monitoring
1	—	12.5	12.5	BP (sitting and standing) should be monitored hourly for 6 hours after taking. Not required if the patient is asleep
2	12.5	12.5	25	BP (sitting and standing), pulse, temperature, respiratory rate before the morning dose and repeated 2 and 6 hours after the dose
3	12.5	25	37.5 (a)	FBC due (WBCs, neutrophils, eosinophils) BP (sitting and standing), pulse, temperature, respiratory rate before the morning dose and repeated 6 hours after the dose
4	25	25	50	BP (sitting and standing), pulse, temperature, respiratory rate before the morning dose and repeated 6 hours after the dose
5	25	50	75	As for day 4
6	50	50	100	As for day 4
7	50	50	100	As for day 4
8	50	75	125	FBC due (WBCs, neutrophils, eosinophils), monitor for sedation, constipation, hypersalivation, troponin T or I and C-reactive protein. Other parameters as for day 4
9	75	75	150	As for day 4
10	75	100	175	As for day 4
11	100	100	200	As for day 4
12	100	125	225	As for day 4
13	125	125	250 (b)	As for day 4
14	125	150	275	As for day 4

Table 4.2: Dosing and monitoring regimen for inpatients *continued*

Day	Morning dose (mg)	Evening dose (mg)*	Total daily dose (mg)	Monitoring
15–17	150	150	300	FBC due (WBCs, neutrophils, eosinophils), monitor for sedation, constipation, hypersalivation, troponin T or I and C-reactive protein. Daily BP (sitting and standing), pulse, temperature, respiratory rate to continue until the dose is stable and no unacceptable adverse effects noted
18–21	150	200	350 (c)	Daily BP (sitting and standing), pulse, temperature, respiratory rate to continue until the dose is stable and no unacceptable adverse effects noted
22–28	200	200	400	As per days 15–17
29–32	200	250	450 (d)	Weight (including BMI, and abdominal circumference), monitor for sedation, constipation and hypersalivation. Assess mental state. Other parameters as per days 18–21
33–36	200	300	500	As per days 15–17
37–40	250	300	550 (e)	As per days 15–17

*Consider giving a larger proportion of the dose in the evening if daytime sedation is a concern

BP = *blood pressure*, FBC = *full blood count*, WBCs = *white blood count*, BMI = *body mass index*
(a) *target dose for drug-induced psychosis in Parkinson's disease*
(b) *target for adult female non-smokers*[10]*/elderly patients with resistant-schizophrenia*
(c) *target for male non-smokers*[10]
(d) *target for female smokers/resistant childhood-onset schizophrenia*[10]
(e) *target for male smokers*[10]

Community/outpatient initiation of clozapine

With intensive support and a coordinated team approach, many patients can be successfully started on clozapine in the community. This may be through a day-care service, clozapine clinic or with an intensive, community mental health team who can visit the patient regularly at home. Patients who are started on clozapine in the community are subject to the same monitoring and regulations as inpatients (see *Table 4.1*). In addition, a risk analysis investigating compliance, illness severity, available support at home, capacity to understand adverse effects and level of engagement should be considered. In general, it is advisable to start clozapine at the beginning of the week when the majority of services are fully available and avoid dose increases during the weekend. *Table 4.3* suggests a dosing and monitoring regimen for outpatient initiation, which is slightly slower than that given for inpatients.

Ongoing physical health monitoring

Ongoing monitoring of physical health is essential for those receiving clozapine. This is usually achieved through a coordinated care plan between primary (specialist mental health services) and secondary care services (general practitioners/family physicians). At every review, patients, family and carers should receive advice on maintaining an active and healthy lifestyle. *Table 4.4* recommends the ongoing physical health monitoring for those receiving clozapine.

Table 4.3: Dosing and monitoring regimen for outpatients[8,9,11]

Day	Morning dose (mg)	Evening dose (mg)*	Total daily dose (mg)	Monitoring (At all times the patient, family and carers should have an emergency number to call in case of adverse effects)
1: Monday	—	12.5	12.5	BP (sitting and standing) should be monitored hourly for 6 hours after taking. Not required if the patient is asleep
2: Tuesday	12.5	12.5	25	BP (sitting and standing), pulse, temperature, respiratory rate before the morning dose and repeated 2 and 6 hours after the dose
3: Wednesday	12.5	25	37.5	FBC due (WBCs, neutrophils, eosinophils) BP (sitting and standing), pulse, temperature, respiratory rate before the morning dose and repeated 6 hours after the dose. Consider a medical appointment to review progress
4: Thursday	25	25	50	BP (sitting and standing), pulse, temperature, respiratory rate before the morning dose and repeated 6 hours after the dose
5: Friday	25	37.5	62.5	As for day 4
6: Saturday**	25	37.5	62.5	As for day 4
7: Sunday**	25	37.5	62.5	As for day 4
8: Monday	37.5	37.5	75	FBC due (WBCs, neutrophils, eosinophils), monitor for sedation, constipation, hypersalivation, troponin T or I and C-reactive protein. Other parameters as for day 4
9: Tuesday	37.5	50	87.5	As for day 4
10: Wednesday	50	50	100	As for day 4
11: Thursday	50	62.5	112.5	As for day 4
12: Friday	62.5	62.5	125	As for day 4
13: Saturday**	62.5	62.5	125	As for day 4
14: Sunday**	62.5	62.5	125	As for day 4

Table 4.3: Dosing and monitoring regimen for outpatients *continued*

15: Monday	62.5	75	137.5	FBC due (WBCs, neutrophils, eosinophils), monitor for sedation, constipation, hypersalivation, troponin T or I and C-reactive protein. Daily BP (sitting and standing), pulse, temperature, respiratory rate to continue until the dose is stable and no unacceptable adverse effects noted
16: Tuesday	75	75	150	Daily BP (sitting and standing), pulse, temperature, respiratory rate to continue until the dose is stable and no unacceptable adverse effects noted
17: Wednesday	75	100	175	As per day 16
18: Thursday	100	100	200	As per day 16
19: Friday	100	125	225	As per day 16
20: Saturday**	100	125	225	As per day 16
21: Sunday**	100	125	225	As per day 16
22: Monday	125	125	250	FBC due (WBCs, neutrophils, eosinophils), monitor for sedation, constipation, hypersalivation, troponin T or I and C-reactive protein. Daily BP (sitting and standing), pulse, temperature, respiratory rate to continue until the dose is stable and no unacceptable adverse effects noted
23: Tuesday	125	150	275	As per day 16
24: Wednesday	150	150	300	As per day 16
25: Thursday	150	175	325	As per day 16
26: Friday	175	175	350	As per day 16
27: Saturday**	175	175	350	As per day 16
28: Sunday**	175	175	350	As per days16

*Consider giving a larger proportion of the dose in the evening if daytime sedation is a concern; ** Some centres suspend physical monitoring at weekends when the dose is not being altered

BP = *blood pressure;* BMI = *body mass index;* FBC = *full blood count;* WBC = *white blood count*

Table 4.4: Ongoing physical health monitoring for those receiving clozapine[8,9]

Parameter	1st month only	3rd month only	Every 6 months	Annually
Blood Pressure (sitting and standing)	Frequently in the first month	✓	✓	✓
Pulse	Frequently in the first month	✓	✓	✓

Temperature	Frequently in the first month	✓	✓	✓
Respiratory rate monitoring	Frequently in the first month	Repeat if clinically indicated		
Urea and electrolytes (including eGFR)	–	–	–	✓
Full blood count (WBCs, neutrophils, eosinophils)	As per national/company guidelines			
ECG	Repeat if clinically indicated			
Blood lipids (cholesterol and triglycerides), fasting sample ideally	✓	✓	✓	✓
Weight (including BMI and abdominal circumference)	✓	✓	✓	✓
Plasma glucose (fasting sample ideally)	✓	✓	✓	✓
Liver function tests (ALT, AST, bilirubin, albumin, prothrombin)	✓	✓	–	✓
Troponin T or I	Frequently in the first month	Repeat if clinically indicated		
C-reactive protein	Frequently in the first month	Repeat if clinically indicated		
Monitor for hypersalivation	✓	✓	✓	✓
Monitor for constipation	✓	✓	✓	✓
Monitor for sedation	✓	✓	✓	✓
EEG (Under 16s only)	Repeat if clinically indicated			
Clozapine plasma level	Measure once maintenance dose achieved, repeat if clinically indicated			

ALT = *alanine aminotransferase;* AST = *aspartate aminotransferase;* ECG = *electrocardiogram;* eGFR = *estimated glomerular Filtration rate;* EEG = *electroencephalogram*

Switching from another antipsychotic

Ideally, all antipsychotics should be discontinued before starting clozapine. In practice, however, switching strategies are largely dependent on the patient's mental state and risk of relapse. A more pragmatic approach is to slowly withdraw (by reducing the dose by 20–25% every week) the previous oral antipsychotic while cautiously introducing clozapine. Many antipsychotics share adverse effects with clozapine (e.g. olanzapine — weight gain and sedation, chlorpromazine — sedation and hypotension), so care is needed to monitor and avoid additive effects. Women on antipsychotics which can raise prolactin (e.g. haloperidol, risperidone, amisulpride) and thus impair fertility, need to be advised about adequate contraception and that fertility may return when switching to clozapine. In addition, antipsychotics which are known to prolong the QT interval (e.g. haloperidol, ziprasidone, sertindole etc) will need close ECG monitoring when clozapine is added. All antipsychotic long-acting injections should be stopped before clozapine is started[9], although their therapeutic and adverse effects will continue for several months after the last injection.

Non-adherence with clozapine

Full adherence to long-term medication is generally low, with studies suggesting that less than half of all medication prescribed is taken as recommended[12]. Non-adherence to antipsychotics in schizophrenia is associated with more frequent relapses, admissions to hospital and poorer outcomes[13]. There are many causes of non-adherence and understandably, many people will be reluctant to tell their clinician the full extent or reason for non-adherence. NICE provides guidance on how to involve patients in decisions about their medication and support adherence[14]. The core principles are being non-judgemental, exploring the patient's beliefs about medication, giving them the opportunity to be involved in the decision-making and addressing concerns in an open and appropriate way. Although there is rarely a simple remedy to non-adherence, keeping the medication regimen simple, using reminder cards or prompts (e.g. compliance aids) and backing up information with appropriate written guidance may help[12, 14].

Sporadic adherence with clozapine poses specific problems which need to be highlighted to the patient, family and carers. Perhaps uniquely among antipsychotics, even partial non-adherence to clozapine usually results in prompt return of symptoms.

Figure 4.1: Symptoms associated with the abrupt withdrawal of clozapine[15, 17]

Rapid onset of psychosis (usually occurs with 1–2 days of stopping clozapine)
- Paranoid delusions
- Hallucinations
- Hostility

Cholinergic rebound (varies in severity, often mild and self-limiting)
- Headache
- Nausea/vomiting
- Diarrhoea
- Diaphoresis
- Restlessness

Others (described in case reports)
- Catatonia[22]
- Exacerbation of extrapyramidal symptoms (e.g. dystonias and dyskinesias)[23]
- Delirium[24]
- Insomnia[25]

Abrupt clozapine withdrawal

Sudden withdrawal of clozapine is associated with a rapid onset psychosis (or 'supersensitivity psychosis'), a cholinergic rebound syndrome and other symptoms related to clozapine's receptor binding (*Figure 4.1*).

The incidence of the rapid-onset of psychosis appears to be around 20%, with a typical presentation of 1–2 days[15] following abrupt withdrawal. Those on a higher dose of clozapine appear to be at most risk of withdrawal complications[16]. Worryingly, some authors report the severity of psychotic symptoms after clozapine withdrawal exceeds that recorded before clozapine initiation[15,17]. The cholinergic rebound symptoms vary in severity from mild, self-limiting symptoms of nausea and headache, to more pronounced vomiting and sweating[18]. Anticholinergics such as trihexylphenidyl[19] or other antipsychotics may reduce some but not all of the discontinuation symptoms[20]. Cyproheptadine (a non-selective serotonin receptor antagonists) has also demonstrated some success in reducing clozapine discontinuation symptoms in a case series[21]. Why clozapine causes more pronounced problems on withdrawal than other antipsychotics is unclear. Hypothesises include a dopamine, serotonin or acetylcholine receptor supersensitivitiy, or a long-term pharmacodynamic brain adaption which is revealed only when treatment is removed[15]. It is also likely that the short half-life of clozapine (mean 14.2 hours)[9], which results in a rapid reduction in plasma levels, is a contributing factor, along with the fact that clozapine is often used for the most unwell patients.

Missing 48 hours or more of clozapine

Along with the rapid decline in plasma levels upon clozapine discontinuation, tolerability to adverse effects rapidly falls away. Patients who have missed clozapine for 48 hours or more (taken from the last dose given) should be gradually re-titrated from 12.5mg per day (*Table 4.1* or *4.2*)[9]. The speed of the titration depends on the original acceptance and tolerability of clozapine and can often be more rapid than the original titration. Hypotension, tachycardia and seizures are particular risks when re-starting clozapine but so is relapse, so re-titration should be as rapid as possible. Depending on how long clozapine is missed, the frequency of FBC monitoring may need adjusting (*Table 4.5*).

Planned withdrawal of clozapine

Treatment with clozapine must be discontinued immediately in the event of a life-threatening adverse reaction such as neutropenia, agranulocytosis, myocarditis, cardiomyopathy or liver failure. For those who are planning to come off clozapine (ideally with the agreement of the healthcare team), the dose should be gradually reduced over at least 1–2 weeks to reduce the risk of discontinuation symptoms[9]. Longer withdrawal periods have not been formally investigated but may be beneficial.

Enforcing clozapine

Successful long-term treatment of clozapine requires active engagement and consent from those receiving treatment. Unfortunately, in psychiatry there are occasions where those detained or subject to supervised community treatment refuse consent despite specialist advice. In this situation, the subject of enforcing a trial of clozapine can arise. This should be considered as a last resort and all alternatives such as using clozapine liquid, negotiating compliance with rewards and fully exploring why the individual refuses to consider clozapine should be exhausted first. Psychological interventions and discussions from those already on clozapine can help allay any fears, and often with slow and steady persuasion the patient may accept treatment[26]. Enforcing clozapine and the required venepuncture can have grave consequences for the patient's relationship with the healthcare team, and risks the safety of the staff and patient involved (through needle-stick injury). Theoretically, following an enforced trial of clozapine the patient may gain a degree of insight and voluntarily continue with treatment. However, there are no outcome studies supporting this stance. The Care Quality Commission (CQC) (England only) has provided legal guidance which allows clozapine administration and the associated venepuncture to be performed if necessary under the Mental Health Act, 1983 section 63, without the patient's consent[27], and this has occasionally been reported in practice[28, 29]. The argument for enforcing clozapine may be slightly more convincing in those who have previously shown a good response to clozapine and pose a significant risk of harm to themselves and others[26]. In all potential cases, a second opinion specialist doctor and the views of the full multidisciplinary team must be sought.

There are two published case reports on using intramuscular clozapine to enforce treatment in a forensic psychiatric setting. However, the authors conclude that this is not a long-term viable solution because of global supply problems[30]. Individually prepared injections from hospital sterile production units are another option.

Table 4.5. Guidance from UK manufacturers on the frequency of blood testing following clozapine withdrawal[10] (FBC = *full blood count*)

FBC monitoring frequency before clozapine withdrawal	Off clozapine for less than 48 hours	Off > 48 hours but < 7 days	Off > 7 days	
Weekly	No change to blood monitoring frequency. Continue as normal	No change to monitoring frequency. Re-titration dose as per initial titration	Restart at 18 weeks weekly monitoring. Re-titration dose as for initial titration	
FBC Monitoring frequency before clozapine withdrawal	**Off <48 hours**	**Off > 48 hours but < 4 days**	**Off > 4 days but < 28 days**	**Off > 28 days**
Fortnightly and monthly	No change to monitoring frequency. Continue as normal	No change to monitoring frequency. Re-titration dose as per initial titration	Weekly for 6 weeks and then back to previous monitoring frequency	To restart at 18 weeks weekly monitoring. Re-titration dose as for initial titration

Summary

- Before starting clozapine, patients should undergo a thorough physical health review and any previous health complaints should be investigated. This should include a full assessment for potential drug or herbal interactions.
- Many adverse effects of clozapine are predictable, dose dependent and often related to the speed of titration.
- The safe use of clozapine is dependent on a slow, cautious titration with much emphasis on physical health monitoring.
- Those starting clozapine in the community are subject to the same intensive monitoring and regulations as inpatients.
- Abrupt withdrawal of clozapine can lead to a rapid-onset psychosis and other discontinuation symptoms.
- Those receiving clozapine should be counselled on risks of sudden withdrawal and be engaged in open and non-judgemental discussions on adherence.
- Stopping clozapine for more than 48 hours requires a re-titration of the dose, usually at a faster rate than in naive patients.

References

1. Mistry H, Osborn D. Underuse of clozapine in treatment-resistant schizophrenia. *Adv Psychiatr Treatment* 2011; **17:** 250–5
2. National Collaborating Centre for Mental Health. *Schizophrenia: Core Interventions in the Treatment of Schizophrenia in Adults in Primary and Secondary Care* (Updated Edition) (NICE Clinical Guideline CG82). National Institute for Health and Clinical Excellence, 2009
3. Howes O, Vergunst F, Gee S, McGuire P, Kapur S, Taylor D. Adherence to treatment guidelines in clinical practice: study of antipsychotic treatment prior to clozapine initiation. *Br J Psychiatry* 2012; **201:** 481–5
4. Wheeler A. Treatment pathway and patterns of clozapine prescribing for schizophrenia in New Zealand. *Ann Pharmacother* 2008; **42:** 852–60
5. Downs J, Zinkler M. Clozapine: National review of postcode prescribing. *Psychiatr Bull* 2007; **31:** 384–7
6. Nielsen J, Dahm M, Lublin H, Taylor D. Psychiatrists' attitude towards and knowledge of clozapine treatment. *J Psychopharmacol* 2010; **24:** 965–71
7. Taylor D, Shapland L, Laverick G, Bond J. Clozapine – a survey of patient perceptions. *Psychiatr Bull* 2000; **24:** 450–2
8. Taylor D, Paton C, Kapur S. *The Maudsley Prescribing guidelines.* 11th edition: Oxford: Wiley-Blackwell: 2012
9. Clozaril specific product characteristics (SPC). Novartis. www.medicines.org.uk (accessed Jan 2013)
10. Rostami-Hodjegan A, Amin A, Spencer E, Lennard M, Tucker G, Flanagan R. Influence of dose, cigarette smoking, age, sex, and metabolic activity on plasma clozapine concentrations: a predictive model and nomograms to aid clozapine dose adjustment and to assess compliance in individual patients. *J Clin Psychopharmacol* 2004; **24:** 70–8
11. O'Brien A. Starting clozapine in the community: a UK perspective. *CNS Drugs* 2004; **18:** 845–52
12. Haynes RB, Ackloo E, Sahota N, McDonald HP, Yao X. Interventions for enhancing medication

adherence. Cochrane Database of Systematic Reviews 2008, Issue 2. Art. No.: CD000011. DOI: 10.1002/14651858.CD000011.pub3

13. Morken G, Widen J, Grawe K. Non-adherence to antipsychotic medication, relapse and rehospitalisation in recent onset-schizophrenia. *BMC Psychiatry* 2008; **8:** 32

14. National Collaborating Centre for Primary Care. *Medicines adherence. Involving patients in decisions about prescribed medication and supporting adherence.* (NICE Clinical Guideline CG76). National Institute for Health and Clinical Excellence, 2009.

15. Moncrieff J. Does antipsychotic withdrawal provoke psychosis? Review of the literature on rapid onset psychosis (supersensitivity psychosis) and withdrawal-related relapse. *Acta Psychiatrica Scand* 2006; **114:** 3–13

16. Durst R, Teitelbaum A, Katz G, Knobler H. Withdrawal from clozapine: The 'Rebound Phenomen'. *Isr J Psychiatry Relat Sci* 1999; **36:** 122–8

17. Shore D, Matthews S, Cott J, Lieberman JA. Clinical implications of clozapine discontinuation: Report of an NIMH workshop. *Schizophr Bull* 1995; **21:** 333–8

18. Shlovitz T, Welke T, Tigel P, Anand R, Hartman R, Sramek J, et al. Cholinergic rebound and rapid onset psychosis following abrupt clozapine withdrawal. *Schizophr Bull* 1996; **22:** 591–5

19. De Leon J, Stanilla J, White A, Simpson G. Anticholinergics to treat clozapine withdrawal. *J Clin Psychiatry* 1994; **55:** 119–20

20. Seppala N, Kovio C, Leinonen E. Effect of anticholinergics in preventing acute deterioration in patients undergoing abrupt clozapine withdrawal. *CNS Drugs* 2005; **19:** 1049–55

21. Meltzer H, Lee M, Ranian R, Mason E, Cola P. Relapse following clozapine withdrawal: Effect of neuroleptic drugs and cyproheptadine. *Psychopharmacology* 1996; **124:** 176–87

22. Bastiampillai T, Forooziya F, Dhillon R. Clozapine-withdrawal catatonia. *Aust N Z J Psychiatry* 2009; **43:** 283–4

23. Ahmed S, Chengappa K, Naidu V, Baker R, Parepally H, Schooler N. Clozapine withdrawal-emergent dystonias and dyskinesias: A case series. *J Clin Psychiatry* 1998; **59:** 472–7

24. Stanila J, De Leon J, Simpson G. Clozapine withdrawal resulting in delirium with psychosis. A report of three cases. *J Clin Psychiatry* 1997; **58:** 252–5

25. Staedt J, Stoppe G, Hajak G, Ruther E. Rebound insomnia after abrupt clozapine withdrawal. *Eur Arch Psychiatry Clin Neurosci* 1999; **246:** 79–82

26. Barnes T. Commentart: The risks of enforcing clozapine therapy. *Psychiatr Bull* 1999; **23:** 656–7

27. Care Quality Commission. *The Administration of Clozapine and other treatments requiring blood tests under the provision of the Mental Health Act.* Updated 3rd November 2008. http://archive.cqc.org.uk/ (accessed 2 January 2013)

28. Pereira S, Beer D, Paton C. When all else fails. A locally devised structured decision process for enforcing clozapine therapy. *Psychiatr Bull* 1999; **23:** 654–6

29. Pereira S, Beer S, Paton. Enforcing treatment with clozapine: survey of views and practice. *Psychiatr Bull* 1999; **23:** 342–5

30. Kasinathan J, Mastroianni T. Evaluating the use of enforced clozapine in an Australian forensic psychiatric setting: two cases. *BMC Psychiatry* 2007; **7(Suppl 1):** 13

5. Adverse reactions

5.1: Haematological effects

Neutropenia and agranulocytosis

Clozapine can cause a number of blood dyscrasias. Neutropenia and agranulocytosis are the best recognised and are the reason for mandatory monitoring in most countries. Neutropenia is defined as a neutrophil count of 0.5–1.5x109/L, agranulocytosis as a neutrophil count of less than 0.5 x109/L[1]. The overall incidence of neutropenia is around 2.7% and agranulocytosis is between 0.7 and 0.8%[2,3]. The peak incidence of both occurs between 6–18 weeks of clozapine treatment[2] and the risk considerably declines after the first year. The second year incidence rate is quoted in one study as 0.7% for neutropenia and 0.07% for agranulocytosis[2]; an incidence similar to that seen with the phenothiazines[4]. Both neutropenia and agranulocytosis are generally reversible on discontinuation of clozapine. With close monitoring of white blood cells (WBCs), there have only been four deaths reported from agranulocytosis in the UK[5]. These reactions appear idiosyncratic with no correlation to the dose of clozapine. However, a number of risk factors for developing blood dyscrasias have been suggested (*Table 5.1.1*).

Table 5.1.1: Summary of neutropenia and agranulocytosis

	Neutrophil count definition	Overall incidence	Peak incidence	Possible risk factors
Neutropenia	0.5–1.5 x109/L	2.7%	6–18 weeks (49% of cases are reported in this time frame)	Africans and Afro-Caribbeans Low baseline WBC counts Concurrent valproic acid*[13]
Agranulocytosis	Less than 0.5x109/L	0.7–0.8%	6–18 weeks (82% of cases are reported in this time frame)	Female[3] Older age Asian race[2] Ashkenazic Jews The single nucleotide polymorphism, HLA-DQB1 6672G>C

* = Unclear significance, often combined with clozapine

Intriguingly, genetic studies point to variations in the human leukocyte antigen system (HLAs) as having a role in increasing susceptibility to clozapine-induced agranulocytosis[6]. A specific variant (6672G>C) in HLA-DQB1 has recently been associated with an increased risk of clozapine-induced agranulocytosis (by 16.9 times[7]). Identification of this specific variant may prove a useful tool to help mitigate some of the risks when considering a re-challenge with clozapine following neutropenia[8].

The exact mechanism of clozapine-induced neutropenia and agranulocytosis is unclear. In agranulocytosis the cells affected are the neutrophil precursor cells and mature peripheral neutrophils. In neutropenia, only the peripheral neutrophils appear affected[9]. Several theories exist which point either to a potentially toxic clozapine metabolite (e.g. a reactive nitrenium ion), or an immune-mediated response[9]. Loeffler et al reported an increased apoptosis of blood neutrophils in a 45-year-old woman who developed clozapine-induced agranulocytosis five weeks into treatment[10]. In this case report, they found an enhanced expression of the pro-apoptotic proteins Bax and Bik and a decrease of the anti-apoptotic protein BCl-XLmRNA and speculated this may have occurred because of a reactive nitrenium ion or oxidative stress[10]. Note however, transient neutropenia (where values return to normal with continued clozapine) may occur[9] and there are case reports of a diurnal variation in neutrophil count, where higher neutrophil counts are found in the afternoon[11].

In most countries (*Appendix 1*), the clozapine manufacturers have developed a robust monitoring service which records WBC counts before clozapine can be supplied. A colour-coded system for results is often used to highlight those patients who should stop clozapine because of neutropenia, or who require extra monitoring (*Table 5.1.2*).

Table 5.1.2: Blood results coloured-coded system (UK, US, Canada)

Colour	WBC count 10x9/L	Neutrophil count 10x9/L	Action
Green	>3.5	>2.0	Nil continue
Amber	3.0–3.5	1.5–2.0	Twice-weekly full blood counts
Red	<3.0	<1.5	Stop clozapine and repeat the blood count to confirm the result

Many companies also highlight to the treating clinician when the lowest normal result (or lowest green to date) is recorded so extra monitoring and vigilance can be instigated. Of course, these reference ranges are derived from white populations and may not reflect commonly occurring values in other ethnic groups.

Benign ethnic neutropenia (BEN)

BEN occurs approximately in 25–50% of people of African descent and has also been reported in Jewish, Middle Eastern and Afro-Caribbean groups[12]. Although it is the most common cause of neutropenia, it has not been associated with agranulocytosis or any other symptom suggesting an impaired immune system. BEN is thought to occur because mature granulocytes are retained in the marrow storage pool, rather than being released to the peripheral circulation[12]. Since 2002 in the UK, the recognition of BEN has led to the amendment of the clozapine monitoring blood counts following a written, confirmed diagnosis by a haematologist (*Table 5.1.3*). While this has improved access to clozapine, it still remains underutilised in black patients[13].

Table 5.1.3: Blood results coloured-coded system for those diagnosed with BEN (UK)

Colour	WBC count 10x9/L	Neutrophil count 10x9/L	Action
Green	>3.0	>1.5	Nil continue
Amber	2.5–3.0	1.0–1.5	Twice-weekly full blood counts
Red	<2.5	<1.0	Stop clozapine and repeat the blood count to confirm the result

Rechallenging clozapine following neutropenia or agranulocytosis

The decision to restart clozapine following an episode of neutropenia should only be undertaken with extreme caution and based on a thorough case by case assessment of the risks and potential benefits. Where there is a clear episode of agranulocytosis caused by clozapine, a rechallenge is not usually considered appropriate. If there were additional risk factors for developing neutropenia (such as a drug interaction or medical comorbidity), this should be resolved first. In one study of 53 patients rechallenged with clozapine following a confirmed blood dyscrasia, 20 (38%) experienced a further episode[15]. The second episode generally occurred quicker (median time 5.5 weeks), was more severe and lasted longer than the first blood dyscrasia[15]. Most worryingly, of these 20 patients, nine (45%) developed full-blown agranulocytosis upon the rechallenge (in these nine, the first episode of blood dyscrasia was neutropenia). This represented a 22-fold increase in the risk of agranulocytosis in the rechallenge group compared with clozapine-naïve patients[15].

Role of lithium in managing clozapine-induced neutropenia

Lithium increases neutrophil count (mean increase 2×10^9/l) both acutely and chronically[16], and has occasionally been used to prevent and treat clozapine-induced neutropenia in both adults and children[16, 17]. It is most often used to increase neutrophils in BEN to allow the use of clozapine. A minimum serum lithium level of 0.4mmol/l may be required to achieve this increase, which is thought to be caused by an upregulation of granulopoiesis-stimulating factors[18]. White cells are fully formed and function normally and the neutrophil count appears to increase rapidly over the first week of lithium administration[18]. However, the use of lithium is not without risk. Lithium does not prevent true clozapine-induced agranulocytosis and there is concern that lithium may mask impending agranulocytosis[17]. There is also one case of fatal agranulocytosis with the combination of lithium and clozapine and another case where the bone marrow was resistant to treatment with GM-CSF[16]. Other adverse reactions reported with this combination include neuroleptic malignant syndrome (NMS), diabetic ketoacidosis and reversible neurotoxicity[19].

Use of granulocyte colony stimulating factor (G-CSF)

Filgrastim (human G-CSF) has been used in several case reports to shorten the duration of clozapine-induced agranulocytosis (recovery time is shortened by around 50%)[9, 20]. There are also a few published cases of longer term treatment with filgrastim to allow continued clozapine use despite neutropenia[9, 21, 22]. There are also however, two published cases where repeated filgrastim use failed to reverse clozapine-induced agranulocytosis[21, 23]. One or two specialist centres in the UK do use long-term GCS-F, but in conjunction with guidance from a haematologist. Without more evidence of the safety, efficacy and dosing regimen, such long-term treatment should be avoided.

Eosinophillia

Eosinophilia (>0.7×10^9/L[3]) is commonly seen with clozapine — an incidence of around 13%[22] (although rates of up to 62% have been reported[25]). Eosinophilia generally occurs in the first four weeks of treatment, usually resolves spontaneously without intervention and may occur more frequently in women[26]. In the majority of cases clozapine-induced eosinophilia is benign, but there are occasional reports linking this blood dyscrasia with eosinophilic cardiomyopathy[24]. As a result of this possible association, manufacturers of clozapine recommend that clozapine should be discontinued if eosinophil count rises above 3.0×10^9/L and should not be restarted until the count is below 1×10^9/L[27]. There is no strong evidence to link clozapine-induced eosinophilia with any other complication.

Summary

- The peak incidence of neutropenia or agranulocytosis occurs between 6–18 weeks of clozapine treatment.
- Agranulocytosis is life-threatening and clozapine must be immediately discontinued.
- All patients receiving clozapine should be regularly reminded to contact their doctor or healthcare team should any signs of infection develop (such as flu-like complaints, fever or sore throat).

- The decision to restart clozapine following an episode of neutropenia should only be undertaken with extreme caution and based on a thorough case by case assessment of the risks and potential benefits.
- Future blood dyscrasias usually occur quicker, are more severe and last longer than the first episode.
- Although both lithium and filgrastim have been used to elevate WBCs following clozapine-induced neutropenia, both treatments carry significant risk and cannot be recommended routinely.
- Eosinophilia is commonly reported in the first four weeks of clozapine treatment and usually resolves spontaneously without treatment. It may be linked to myocarditis.

Further reading

Whiskey E, Taylor D. Restarting clozapine after neutropenia. Evaluating the possibilities and practicalities. *CNS Drugs* 2007; **21:** 25–35

References

1. Atkin K, Kendall F, Gould D, Freeman H, Lieberman J, O'Sullivan D. Neutropenia and Agranulocytosis in patients receiving clozapine in the UK and Ireland. *Br J Psychiatry* 1996; **169:** 483–8
2. Munro J, O'Sullivan D, Andrews C, Arana A, Mortimer A, Kerwin R. Active monitoring of 12,760 clozapine recipients in the UK and Ireland. *Br J Psychiatry* 1999; **175:** 576–80
3. Alvir JMJ, Lieberman JA, Safferman AZ, Schwimmer JL, Schaaf JA. Clozapine-induced agranulocytosis: Incidence and risk factors in the United States. *N Engl J Med* 1993; **329:** 162–7
4. Mandel A, Gross M. Agranulocytosis and phenothiazines. *Dis Nervous System* 1968; **29:** 32–6
5. Medicines and Healthcare products regulatory Authority. Drug Analysis Prints (DAP) Clozapine. http://www.mhra.gov.uk (accessed 20 February 2012)
6. Opgen-Rhein C, Dettling M. Clozapine induced agranulocytosis and its genetic determinants. *Pharmacogenomics* 2008; **9:** 1101–11
7. Athanasiou MC, Dettling M, Cascorbi I, Mosyagin I, Salisbury BA, Pierz KA, et al. Candidate gene analysis identifies a polymorphism in HLA-DQB1 associated with clozapine induced agranulocytosis. *J Clin Psychiatry* 2011; **72:** 458–63
8. McKnight C, Guirgis H, Votolato N. Clozapine rechallenge after excluding the high risk clozapine induced agranulocytosis genotype of HLA-DQB1 6672G>C. *Am J Psychiatry* 2011; **168:** 1120
9. Whiskey E, Taylor D (2007) Restarting clozapine after neutropenia. Evaluating the possibilities and practicalities. *CNS Drugs* 2007; **21:** 25–35.
10. Loeffler S, Fehsel K, Henning U, Fischer J, Agelink M, Kolb-Bachofen V, et al. Increased apoptosis of neutrophils in a case of clozapine-induced agranulocytosis. *Pharmacopsychiatry* 2003; **36:** 37–41
11. Spina SP, Corrigan SP. Continuing clozapine therapy despite morning pseudoneutropenia. *Can J Hosp Pharmacy* 2007; **60:** 260–4
12. Shoenfeld Y, Alkan M, Aslay A, Carmeli Y, Katz M (1988) Benign familial leukopenia and neutropenia in different ethnic groups. *Eur J Haematol* 1988; **41:** 273–7

13. Whiskey E, Olofinjana O, Taylor D. The importance of the recognition of benign ethnic neutropenia in black patients during treatment with clozapine: case reports and database study. *J Psychopharmacol* 2011; **25:** 842–5
14. Ratanajamit C, Musakopas C. Vasiknanonte S, Reanmongkol W. Incidence and risk for neutropenia/agranulocytosis among clozapine users: A retrospective cohort study. *Int J Psychiatry Clin Practice* 2010; **14:** 109–15
15. Dunk L, Annan L, Andrew C. Rechallenge with clozapine following leucopenia or neutropenia during previous therapy. *Br J Psychiatry* 2006; **188:** 255–63
16. Paton C, Esop R. Managing clozapine-induced neutropenia with lithium. *Psychiatr Bull* 2005; **29:** 186–8
17. Kanaan R, Kerwin R. Lithium and clozapine rechallenge: A retrospective case analysis. *J Clin Psychiatry* 2006; **67:** 756–60
18. Esposito D, Rouillon F, Limosin F. Continuing clozapine treatment despite neutropenia. *Eur J Clin Pharmacol* 2005; **60:** 759–64.
19. Bazire S. *Psychotropic Drug Directory 2012*. Lloyd-Reinhold Communications LLP, Stratford-upon-Avon
20. Harris S, Mattox B. Clozapine-rechallenge resulting in agranulocytosis: Treatment with granulocyte colony-stimulating factor (G-CSF). *J Pharm Practice* 2010; **23:** 183
21. Joffe G, eskelinen S, Sailas E. Add on filgrastim during clozapine rechallenge in patients with a history of clozapine-related granulocytopenia/agranulocytosis. *Am J Psychiatry* 2009; **166:** 236
22. Mattewson K, Lindenmayer J. Clozapine and granulocyte-stimulating factor: Potential for long-term combination treatment for clozapine-induced neutropenia. *J Clin Psychopharmacol* 2007; **27:** 714–15
23. Stewart J, Majczenko T. Failure of filgrastim to prevent severe clozapine induced agranulocytosis. *South Med J* 2008; **101:** 639–40
24. Chatterton R. Eosinophilia after commencement of clozapine treatment. *Aust N Z J Psychiatry* 1997; **31:** 874–6
25. Hummer M, Kurz M, Barnas C, Saria A, Fleichhacker W. Clozapine induced transient white blood count disorders. *J Clin Psychiatry* 1994; **55:** 429–32
26. Banov M, Tohen M, Friedberg J. High risk of eosinophilia in women treated with clozapine. *J Clin Psychiatry* 1993; **54:** 466–9
27. Clozaril specific product characteristics (SPC). www.medicines.org.uk (accessed13 March 2012)

5.2: Diabetes mellitus

Diabetes mellitus is a complex and progressive metabolic disorder, which is associated with an increased risk of cardiovascular disease and is thought to reduce life expectancy by up to seven years[1]. Approximately 1.9 million people in the UK (3.5–5% of the population) have diabetes and there may be a further 0.5 million who are undiagnosed[1]. Impaired glucose tolerance (a pre-diabetic state) may be 2–3 times more common than diabetes[2]. Complications of diabetes include cardiovascular and cerebrovascular disease, renal disease, ocular defects (including blindness), neuropathic pain and erectile dysfunction[1]. The definition of diabetes and common symptoms from the World Health Organization (WHO) are given in *Figures 5.2.1* and *5.2.2*.

Figure 5.2.1: Definition of diabetes[3]

Diabetes
Fasting plasma glucose ≥7.0mmol/l (126mg/dl) OR
2–h plasma glucose ≥11.1mmol/l (200mg/dl)

Impaired glucose tolerance (IGT)
Fasting plasma glucose<7.0mmol/l (126mg/dl) AND
2–h plasma glucose ≥7.8 and <11.1mmol/l
(140mg/dl and 200mg/dl)

Impaired fasting glucose (IFG)
Fasting plasma 6.1 to 6.9mmol/l (110–125mg/dl)
and glucose 2–h plasma glucose (if measured)
<7.8mmol/l (140mg/dl)

Figure 5.2.2: Common symptoms associated with diabetes[4]

- Polyuria
- Polydipsia
- Constant hunger
- Weight loss
- Fatigue
- Vision changes

Type 1 diabetes (10–15% of diabetes cases) is characterised by a deficient insulin production and requires daily insulin injections. Symptoms may occur suddenly

Type 2 diabetes (85–90% of diabetes cases) is associated with insulin insensitivity and excessive bodyweight. Symptoms are often less marked and associated with a more gradual onset

Schizophrenia and diabetes

People with schizophrenia have a higher rate of diabetes than the general population and this observation pre-dates the widespread use of antipsychotics[5, 6]. Sir Henry Maudsley, in *The Pathology of Mind* (1880) wrote[7]: 'Diabetes is a disease which often shows itself in families in which insanity prevails'.

The prevalence rate of diabetes in those with schizophrenia is around 15% or 2–3 times the risk in the general population[5, 6]. The reason for this is unclear, but it is most likely to be a combination of factors. Some authors have suggested that there is a direct genetic link with shared susceptible genes[8], while others have pointed to environmental factors which are exacerbated in those with schizophrenia (*Figure 5.2.3*)[5].

Figure 5.2.3: Factors influencing the risk of diabetes in people with schizophrenia[5,9]

Choice of atypical (unknown risk),
Olanzapine and clozapine
are the most likely to cause diabetes

Atypical vs typical (relative risk of 1.32)

Schizophrenia (200–300% increased risk)
(May predispose to factors below, e.g. inactivity, poor self-care)

Environmental and genetic risk factors (most influence)

- Family history of diabetes (first degree relative with diabetes)
- Poor diet (High fat, low fibre, poor fruit and vegetables intake)
- Inactivity
- Poor fetal growth
- Low birth weight/prematurity
- Obesity/high body mass index (BMI)
- Increasing age (risk of diabetes increases above 45 years)
- Lipid level abnormalities
- Ethnicity (non-Caucasian)
- Gender (men are at a higher risk of type 2 diabetes)

Antipsychotics and diabetes

Both first and second generation antipsychotics have been associated with changes in glucose levels and an increased risk of diabetes[9, 10]. Second generation antipsychotics have demonstrated a small increased risk for diabetes versus first generation drugs (relative risk was 1.32, 95% CI 1.15–1.51)[11] and olanzapine and clozapine appear to show the greatest elevations in glucose levels[12,13] and risk of diabetes[14]. However, compared with genetic and environmental risk factors (*Figure 5.3*), the increased risk from olanzapine and clozapine is small (hazard ratio for clozapine was 1.57, 95% CI 1.31–1.89, olanzapine was 1.15, 95% CI 1.07–1.24)[14], and may in part be explained by the increased frequency of testing for diabetes[15].

Clozapine and diabetes

In case reports clozapine has been associated with transient hyperglycaemia, diabetes ketoacidosis (including fatalities), new onset diabetes mellitus and exacerbation of pre-existing diabetes[16]. Although clozapine appears to have the strongest association with the risk of diabetes[17, 18], whether it is significantly worse than other antipsychotics is contested[10, 19–21]. Diabetes with clozapine can occur at any time, although over half of all cases are reported in the first three months of therapy[22]. Diabetes does not appear to be related to the dose of clozapine[22] and can occur independently of weight gain[16, 23]. Ethnicity (non-Caucasian) and previous family history of diabetes appear to increase the risk of clozapine-related diabetes[16, 23].

In naturalistic studies of clozapine patients, the cumulative incidence of new-onset diabetes with clozapine was reported to be 37% at five years (n=82)[24] and 43% at 10 years (n=96)[23].

Clozapine and ketoacidosis

There are many case reports linking clozapine to diabetic ketoacidosis[25–28], including a number of fatalities[22, 29]. Ketoacidosis with clozapine is often reported in those with no history of diabetes and does not appear to be related to the dose or duration of clozapine treatment[28]. Ketoacidosis can be quickly fatal so any suspected cases should prompt immediate medical attention and cessation of clozapine. Having multiple medical problems at the time of the ketoacidosis appears to increase the risk of death[22]. Whether clozapine can be re-introduced following ketoacidosis is unclear. Many cases report an immediate increase in serum glucose when clozapine is restarted following ketoacidosis[25] or new-onset diabetes[22]. All clinicians should be alert to this potential complication (*Figure 5.2.4*).

Underlying mechanism behind clozapine and diabetes

The mechanism behind clozapine increasing the risk of diabetes is unclear and probably multifactorial. Clozapine is known to be a potent histamine1 receptor antagonist which may stimulate hypothalamic AMP-protein kinase (AMPK)[31]. AMPK stimulates catabolic and anabolic pathways, which regulate energy balance and enhance appetite[31]. In animal studies, histamine$_1$ receptor antagonism has also been shown to impair leptin responsiveness (an endogenous anorexigenic peptide) and cause weight gain[31]. Serotonin 2C antagonism (seen with clozapine and its metabolites) has also been associated with chronic hyperphagia and associated obesity and hyperinsulinaemia[32]. Weight gain has an established link with causing type 2 diabetes[1], but in light of many studies being unable to demonstrate a link between weight gain and clozapine-related diabetes, it is likely to be but one part of the picture[5]. In further animal studies, clozapine has been shown to inhibit glucose transport (via pheochromocytoma cells)[33] and reduce electrical activity across pancreatic β-cells[34].

Treatment and monitoring for clozapine-induced diabetes

Reducing the risk of clozapine-related diabetes and its associated complications begins with appropriate and timely monitoring of blood glucose (*Chapter 4*). Before

Figure 5.2.4: Signs and symptoms associated with diabetic ketoacidosis[30]

- Polyurea/polydypsia
- Elevated blood glucose (>11mmol/L)
- Acidaemia (<pH 7.3)
- Hyper-osmolarity
- Serum and urine ketones
- Smell of ketones on breath
- Lethargy/drowsiness
- Dehydration
- Abdominal pain
- Hyperventilation
- Hypothermia
- Confusion
- Nausea/vomiting

initiating clozapine, patients should have a fasting blood glucose test performed and be fully investigated for any family or personal history of diabetes[35]. Fasting blood glucose tests should be repeated after the first and third months of clozapine therapy, then regularly every six or twelve months depending on the presence of risk factors (e.g. weight gain or family history). If a fasting blood glucose is not acceptable to the patient, a urine glucose and or random plasma glucose are still useful particularly alongside HbA_{1C} levels. Although various national guidelines recommend close glucose monitoring in all patients receiving antipsychotics[35, 36], monitoring still appears to be suboptimal[37, 38]. At every opportunity (or at least annually) the patient, family or carers should be offered advice on a healthy diet, active lifestyle and the importance of maintaining blood glucose and blood pressure within the normal range[1]. In addition, patients should be asked to look out for any signs and symptoms of diabetes (*Figure 5.2.2*).

Few people with type 2 diabetes are adequately controlled by simply making dietary changes and most will require drug intervention and specialist advice. Metformin is usually considered the treatment of choice for type 2 diabetes, followed by a sulfonylurea[1]. In the majority of cases of clozapine-related diabetes, with appropriate treatment for hyperglycaemia clozapine treatment can continue[22].

There is a small (n=18) 8-week RCT investigating rosiglitazone for clozapine-induced hyperglycaemia and, although not statistically significant, rosiglitazone demonstrated a trend towards an improvement[39]. However, rosiglitazone is no longer marketed in the European Union and is subject to restricted use in the US due to concerns over increased risk of myocardial infarctions[40]. Modafinil failed to show any improvements of plasma glucose in clozapine patients (n=35, 8-week RCT)[41] and pioglitazone[42] and orlistat[43] may improve clozapine-induced hyperglycaemia, but no formal studies have been conducted.

Summary

- In naturalistic studies the rates of new-onset diabetes mellitus with clozapine were 37% at five years and 43% at 10 years.
- Half of all cases of new-onset of diabetes are reported in the first three months of clozapine therapy.

- The diabetes does not appear to be related to the dose of clozapine and can occur independently of weight gain.
- Compared with genetic and environmental risk factors however (age, race, family history, weight), the increased risk from clozapine is small.
- Ketoacidosis can be quickly fatal so any suspected cases should prompt immediate medical attention and cessation of clozapine.
- Before initiating clozapine, patients should have a fasting blood glucose test and be fully investigated for any family or personal history of diabetes.
- Fasting blood glucose should be repeated after the first and third months of treatment, then every six to twelve months depending on risk factors.
- If fasting blood glucose is not acceptable to the patient, a urine glucose and or random plasma glucose are still useful particularly alongside HbA_{1C} levels.
- At every opportunity (or at least annually) the patient, family or carers should be offered advice on a healthy diet, active lifestyle and the importance of maintaining a blood glucose and blood pressure within the normal range.
- In the majority of cases of clozapine-related diabetes, with appropriate treatment for hyperglycaemia (usually metformin), clozapine can continue.

Further reading and resources

Holt R, Peveler R. Association between antipsychotic drugs and diabetes. *Diabetes Obesity Metab* 2006; **8:** 125–35.

http://www.qdscore.org. This site provides a free, type 2 diabetes risk calculation based on extensive data from General Practitioners in England and Wales

References

1. National Collaborating Centre for Chronic Conditions. *Type 2 Diabetes. National clinical guidelines for management in primary and secondary care* (update). (NICE Clinical Guideline CG66). National Institute for Health and Clinical Excellence, 2008
2. Expert Group. Schizophrenia and Diabetes 2003 expert consensus meeting, Dublin 3-4 October 2003: consensus summary. *Br J Psychiatry* 2004; **184(suppl 47):** s112–s114
3. World Health Organization, International Diabetes Federation. *Definition of diabetes mellitus and intermediate hyperglycaemia. Report of a WHO / IDF consultation.* Geneva; WHO: 2006
4. World Health Organization. *Diabetes. Fact sheet No 312.* September 2012. Geneva; World Health Organisation, 2012. Available at: www.who.int.
5. Holt R, Peveler R. Association between antipsychotic drugs and diabetes. *Diabetes, Obesity Metab* 2006; **8:** 125–35
6. Dixon L, Weiden P, Delahanty J, Goldberg R, Postrado L, Lucksted A, et al. Prevalence and correlates of diabetes in National Schizophrenia samples. *Schizophr Bull* 2000; **26:** 903–12
7. Maudsley H. *The Pathology of Mind.* New York. D Appleton and Co, 1880
8. Gough S, O'Donovan M. Clustering of metabolic co-morbidity in schizophrenia: a genetic contribution? *J Psychopharmacol* 2005; **19(Suppl):** 47–55

9. Henderson D. Atypical antipsychotic-induced diabetes mellitus. How strong is the evidence? *CNS Drugs* 2002; **16:** 77–89
10. Lindenmayer J, Czobor P, Volavka J, Citrome L, Sheitman B, McEnvoy J, et al. Changes in glucose and cholesterol levels in patients with schizophrenia and treated with typical or atypical antipsychotics. *Am J Psychiatry* 2003; **160:** 290–6
11. Smith M, Hopkins D, Peveler R, Holt R, Woodward M, Ismail K. First- v. second-generation antipsychotics and risk of diabetes in schizophrenia: systematic review and meta-analysis. *Br J Psychiatry* 2008; **192:** 406–11
12. Newcomer J, Haupt D, Fucetola R, Melson A, Schweiger J, Cooper B, et al. Abnormalities in glucose regulation during antipsychotic treatment of schizophrenia. *Arch Gen Psychiatry* 2002; **59:** 337–45
13. Rummel-Kluge C, Komossa K, Schwarz S, Hunger H, Schmid F, Asenjo C, et al. Head-to-head comparisons of metabolic side effects of second generation antipsychotics in the treatment of schizophrenia: a systematic review and meta-analysis. *Schizophr Res* 2010; **123:** 225–33
14. Leslie D, Rosenheck R. Incidence of newly diagnosed diabetes attributable to atypical antipsychotic medications. *Am J Psychiatry* 2004; **161:** 1709–11
15. Taylor D, Young C, Esop R, Paton C, Walwyn R. Testing for diabetes in hospitalised patients' prescribed antipsychotic drugs. *Br J Psychiatry* 2004; **185:** 152–6
16. Lamberti J, Costea G, Olson D, Crilly J, Maharaj K, Tu X, et al. Diabetes mellitus among outpatients receiving clozapine: Prevalence and Clinical-demographic correlates. *J Clin Psychiatry* 2005; **66:** 900–6
17. Mir S, Taylor D. Atypical antipsychotics and hyperglycaemia. *Int Clin Psychopharmacol* 2001; **16:** 63–74
18. Jin H, Meyer JM, Jeste DV. Phenomenology of and risk factors for new onset diabetes mellitus and diabetic ketoacidosis associated with atypical antipsychotics: an analysis of 45 published cases. *Ann Clin Psychiatry* 2002; **14:** 59–64
19. Schulte P, Bocxe J, Doodeman H, van Haelst I, Cohen D. Risk of new-onset diabetes after long-term treatment with clozapine in comparison to other antipsychotics in patients with schizophrenia. *Eur Psychiatry* 2012; **27:** 0924–9338
20. Lund B, Perry P, Brooks J, Arndt S. Clozapine use in patients with schizophrenia and the risk of diabetes, hyperlipidemia, and hypertension. A claims-based approach. *Arch Gen Psychiatry* 2001; **58:** 1172–76
21. Wang P, Glynn R, Ganz D, Schneeweiss S, Levin R, Avorn J. Clozapine use and risk of diabetes mellitus. *J Clin Psychopharmacol* 2002; **22:** 236–43
22. Koller E, Schneider B, Bennett K, Dubitsky G. Clozapine-associated diabetes. *Am J Med* 2001; **111:** 716–23
23. Henderson D, Nguyen D, Copeland P, Hayden D, Borba C, Louie P, et al. Clozapine, diabetes mellitus, hyperlipidaemia, and cardiovascular risks and mortality: Results of a 10-year naturalistic study. *J Clin Psychiatry* 2005; **66:** 1116–21
24. Henderson D, Cagliero E, Gray C, Nasrallah R, Hayden D, Schoenfeld D et al. Clozapine, diabetes mellitus, weight gain, and lipid abnormalities: A five-year Naturalistic study. *Am J Psychiatry* 2000; **157:** 975–81
25. Colli A, Cocciolo M, Francobandiera G, Rogantin F, Cattalini N. Diabetic ketoacidosis associated with clozapine treatment. *Diabetes Care* 1999; **22:** 176–7
26. Kostakoglu A, Yazici K, Erbas T, Güvener N. Ketoacidosis as a side effect of clozapine: a case report. *Acta Psychiatr Scand* 1997; **93:** 217–18

27. Ali D, Roper T, Riley J. Diabetic ketoacidosis and clozapine. *Postgrad Med J* 1998; **74:** 493
28. Lafayette J, Pirl W, Henderson D. Low-dose clozapine and diabetic ketoacidosis. *Psychosomatics* 2003; **44:** 249–52
29. Wehring H, Kelly D, Love R, Conley R. Deaths from diabetic ketoacidosis after long-tem clozapine treatment. *Am J Psychiatry* 2003; **160:** 2241–2
30. National Collaborating Centre for Women's and Children's health and the National Collaborating Centre for Chronic Conditions. *Type 1 Diabetes. Diagnosis and management of type 1 diabetes in children, young people and adults.* (NICE Clinical Guideline CG15). National Institute for Health and Clinical Excellence, 2004
31. Meltzer H. Illumining the molecular basis for some antipsychotic drug-induced metabolic burden. *Proc Natl Acad Sci U S A* 2007; **104:** 3019–20
32. Stahl S, Mignon L, Meyer J. Which comes first: atypical antipsychotic treatment or cardiometabolic risk? *Acta Psychiatr Scand* 2009; **119:** 171–9
33. Ardizzone T, Bradley R, Freeman A, Dwyer D. Inhibition of glucose transport in PC12 cells by atypical antipsychotics drugs risperidone and clozapine and structural analogs of clozapine. *Brain Res* 2001; **923:** 82–90
34. Best L, Yates A, Reynolds G. Actions of antipsychotic drugs on pancreatic ß-cell function: contrasting effects of clozapine and haloperidol. *J Psychopharmacol* 2005; **9:** 597–601
35. De Hert M, Dekker J, Wood D, Kahl K, Holt R, Möller HJ. Cardiovascular disease and diabetes in people with severe mental illness position statement from the European Psychiatric Association (EPA), supported by the European Association for the Study of Diabetes (EASD) and the European Society of Cardiology (ESC). *Eur Psychiatry* 2009; **24:** 412–24
36. Marder S, Essock S, Miller A, Buchanan R, Casey D, Davis J, et al. Physical health monitoring of patients with schizophrenia. *Am J Psychiatry* 2004; **161:** 1334–49
37. Holt R, Abdelrahman T, Hirsch M, Dhesi Z, George T, Blincoe T, et al. The prevalence of undiagnosed metabolic abnormalities in people with serious mental illness. *J Psychopharmacol* 2010; **24:** 867–73
38. Morrato E, Newcomer J, Kamat S, Baser O, Harnett J, Cuffel B. Metabolic screening after the American Diabetes Association's consensus statement on antipsychotic drugs and diabetes. *Diabetes Care* 2009; **32:** 1037–42
39. Henderson D, Fan X, Sharma B, Copeland P, Borba C, Boxill R, et al. A double-blind, placebo-controlled trial of rosiglitazone for clozapine-induced glucose metabolism impairment in patients with schizophrenia. *Acta Psychiatr Scand* 2009; **119:** 457–65
40. Martindale: *The Complete Drug Reference.* [online] London: Pharmaceutical Press. www.medicinescomplete.com (accessed on 7 January 2013)
41. Henderson D, Freudenreich O, Bora C, Wang X, Copeland P, Macklin E, et al. Effects of modafinil on weight, glucose and lipid metabolism in clozapine-treated patients with schizophrenia. *Schizophr Res* 2011; **130:** 53–6
42. Edinger M, Ebenbichler C, Rettenbacher M, Fleischhacker W. Treatment of antipsychotic-associated hyperglycaemia with pioglitazone: A case series. *J Clin Psychopharmacol* 2007; **27:** 403–4
43. Pavolic Z. Orlistat in the treatment of clozapine-induced hyperglycemia and weight gain. *Eur Psychiatry* 2005; **20:** 52

5.3: Weight gain

Being overweight or obese is a growing worldwide problem and ranks as the fifth leading risk for global deaths[1]. Obesity is associated with an increased risk of diseases which are major causes of morbidity and mortality, such as type 2 diabetes, hypertension, myocardial infarction, stroke, and colon and ovarian cancers[2].

All mental health patients, whether receiving antipsychotics or not should be encouraged to adopt strategies to maintain a healthy weight and an active lifestyle (*Figure 5.3.1*).

Figure 5.3.1: Strategies to help people achieve and maintain a healthy weight[2]

Diet

- Base meals on starchy foods (e.g. potatoes, bread, rice and pasta)
- Eat plenty of fibre-rich foods (e.g. oats, beans, peas, lentils, grains, seeds, fruit and vegetables, wholegrain bread, brown rice and pasta)
- Eat at least five portions of a variety of fruit and vegetables each day
- Eat as little as possible of: fried foods, drinks and confectionery high in added sugars, other food and drinks high in fat and sugar, such as some take-away and fast foods
- Eat breakfast
- Watch the portion size of meals and snacks
- Minimise the calories taken in from alcohol
- Eat a low-fat diet and avoid increasing fat and/or calorie intake
- Drink plenty of fluids (water, milk and fruit juices are the healthiest options). Aim for 1.2L per day or 6–8 glasses a day

Activity

- Make enjoyable activities, such as walking, cycling, swimming, aerobics and gardening, part of everyday life
- Minimise sedentary activities, such as sitting for long periods watching television, at a computer or playing video games
- To maintain good general health aim for at least 30 minutes of moderate intensity physical activity at least five times a week

Body mass index (BMI) and waist circumference are useful measures to assess the risks from being overweight (*Tables 5.3.1, 5.3.2* and *5.3.3*). All people receiving antipsychotics should be encouraged to have their weight, BMI and waist circumference measured regularly.

Table 5.3.1: BMI calculation and interpretation of results[2,3]

BMI = weight (kg)/height $(m)^2$ or BMI = weight (pounds)/height $(in)^2 \times 703$	
Classification	BMI
Healthy weight	18.5–24.9
Overweight	25–29.9
Obesity I	30–34.9
Obesity II	35–39.9
Obesity III	40 or more

Table 5.3.2: Waist circumference interpretation[2]

Classification/recommendation	Waist circumference (cm)	
	Men	Women
Low	<94	<80
High	94–102	80–88
Very high	>102 (~ 40in)	>88 (~ 35in)

Table 5.3.3: Interpretation of BMI and waist circumference results[2]

BMI	Waist circumference			Comorbidities present
	Low	High	Very High	
Overweight				
Obesity I				
Obesity II				
Obesity III				

= General lifestyle advice

= Advice on diet and increasing physical activity

= Advice on diet, increasing physical activity and consider drug intervention

= Advice on diet, increasing physical activity and consider drug or surgical intervention

Clozapine and weight gain

All antipsychotics have been associated with weight gain to a varying degree[4,5,6]. Ziprasidone and aripiprazole appear to cause the least weight gain, while olanzapine and clozapine are consistently associated with the greatest increases[4,5,6]. Clozapine has been shown to cause significantly more weight gain over 10 weeks than most other antipsychotics (the exceptions being chlorpromazine and olanzapine)[6]. The weight gain with antipsychotics is usually rapid in the first 3–4 months and then gradually reaches a plateau with continued use [7,8]. Exactly when this plateau occurs varies with the antipsychotic. With olanzapine and haloperidol, weight stabilises at about nine months of continued use[4,7]. With clozapine however, weight appears to continuously rise for many years. Evidence from meta-analyses and naturalistic studies suggest it may be up to four years before weight stabilises[7,9]. Even once weight has stabilised on clozapine, it may increase again if lifestyle or residential status change dramatically (for example, when long-term residential patients are transferred into independent living)[10].

Figure 5.3.2: Risk factors associated with a larger degree of weight gain with clozapine and other antipsychotics[6]

- Antipsychotic naïve
- Lower BMI before antipsychotic initiated
- A rapid, initial weight gain
- Higher clozapine plasma level — possible association
- Specific genetic variations in the serotonin receptor genes (e.g. the rs3813929 variant of HTR2c) or leptin genes (e.g. the rs7799039, -2548 G/A) are under investigation

The average weight gained and the incidence of weight gain with clozapine vary greatly between studies. Using RCT data, one review suggests the average initial weight gain with clozapine is 1.7kg per month[8]. An early meta-analysis reported the mean weight increase as 4.45kg over 10 weeks[6]. Long-term naturalistic studies report lower rates of weight gain with clozapine and suggest the mean change is from around 3kg over three years[10] (n=174) to 11.6kg over five years (n=82)[9]. Although early reports suggested the frequency of weight gain with clozapine was low (around 4%)[12], more recent reviews suggest more than 20% of all patients experience at least a 10% increase in body weight[8]. Weight gain with clozapine is probably related to dose, or more accurately, plasma levels[13].

It should be noted that the majority of studies report mean weight change at endpoint, which, although useful, disguises the wide variation in weight changes in individuals[4]. Also, for some individuals who are underweight (perhaps because of poor self-care), gaining weight may be a positive aspect of antipsychotic treatment.

Mechanism of action

The mechanism behind clozapine-induced weight gain has been studied in some depth. Of the multiple theories which have been proposed, they are broadly divided into three interacting categories (*Figure 5.3.3*):

- Receptor
- Hormonal
- Genetic influences.

Receptor theories

Clozapine causes both histamine$_1$ (H_1) and serotonin 2C ($5HT_{2C}$) receptor antagonism[14]. H_1 blockade is thought to enhance appetite via the hypothalamic eating centres and activation of AMP kinase[14, 15]. H_1 antagonism has been proposed as the primary mechanism for antipsychotic-induced weight gain[14]. In animal studies, mice with their H_1 receptors knocked out gradually developed obesity through hyperphagia[15]. Obesity and hyperinsulinaemia have also been shown to develop in animal studies where $5HT_{2c}$ receptors have been genetically removed[14]. The combined blockade of both H_1 and $5HT_{2c}$ receptors (as seen with clozapine and olanzapine) may in part explain why these drugs are associated with more weight increases than other antipsychotics.

Hormonal theories

Leptin is a peptide hormone, mainly produced by adipose tissue. It signals to the brain the extent of body fat[16] and is a main regulator of body weight by inducing satiety and stimulating energy expenditure[17]. In general, leptin levels correlate with BMI, percentage of body fat and serum insulin levels. Individuals with obesity tend to have higher leptin levels than those with a normal body weight[16]. While leptin usually alerts the brain to decrease adipose tissue, in obesity (where there are prolonged high leptin levels), leptin resistance in the hypothalamus is thought to develop. This may be through a reduced transport at the blood brain barrier or by leptin receptor abnormalities[16]. Treatment with clozapine has been associated with high circulating leptin levels (or hyperleptinaemia)[17]. This has been postulated to cause leptin resistance such as that seen in obesity[17]. Whether clozapine directly increases leptin or whether the rise is a consequence of other changes (e.g. weight gain or insulin resistance) is unknown[17]. Of interest is that leptin is shown to be regulated by serotoninergic and histaminergic receptors, which may point to the link between clozapine and hyperleptinaemia[17].

Cytokines (such as the tumour necrosis factor alpha, TNF-α) are also involved in body weight regulation and may have a role in antipsychotic weight gain[17], although research is limited at the time of writing.

Genetic theories

There is thought to be a strong genetic influence on weight gain with clozapine. In a study of five monozygotic twins receiving clozapine compared with same-sex siblings, the twins showed a greater similarity in total BMI (heritability estimate of h2=0.8)[18]. Nearly 60 genes have been identified as potentially being involved in antipsychotic weight gain[19]. Of these, genetic variations in the serotonin receptor genes (specifically the rs3813929 variant of HTR_{2c}) and leptin genes (rs7799039, -2548 G/A) have been the most consistently implicated. For an extensive review, see the article by Lett et al listed in further reading.

Despite much advancement in our understanding of weight gain with antipsychotics, how best to modulate these risks remains elusive.

Figure 5.3.3: Proposed mechanisms influencing clozapine-induced weight gain[16, 17, 18, 19]

Receptor theories:

- Histamine$_1$ receptor antagonism
- Serotonin 2c receptor antagonism

Hormonal theories:

- High leptin levels leading to leptin resistance
- Cytokines, e.g. TNF-α involvement

Genetic theories:

- Genetic variations in:
    - Serotonin reception genes
    - Leptin genes
    - Many others proposed (including dopamine, adrenergic and histamine receptor genes)

Does weight gain predict efficacy?

The concept of weight gain with clozapine being a marker of efficacy is intriguing. Short-term studies (<3 months) generally do not show an association between weight gain and clinical effect, but longer trials do report a significant relationship[20]. While it might be considered that the more compliant with clozapine an individual was, the more weight gain and improvement might be expected, there is evidence against this. Meltzer et al closely monitored compliance and plasma levels and still demonstrated that clinical improvement was linked to weight gain[21]. Theories behind this link include a possible involvement of $5HT_{2c}$ receptors in both weight gain and response[21], or a neuroprotective effect from leptin[22].

Treatment of clozapine-induced weight gain

Treatment of weight gain begins with forewarning the individual and active advice on a healthy lifestyle and diet (perhaps with the help of a dietician or personal trainer). There is evidence that individuals with a psychotic disorder benefit from nutritional and physical health advice[23], and that preventative educational interventions can reduce subsequent weight gain with antipsychotics[24,25,26]. Monitoring of weight, BMI and abdominal circumference should be completed at baseline, then repeated at least monthly for the first three months of clozapine treatment (*Chapter 4*). If preventative measures have not been successful, a calorie-restricted diet combined with increased physical activity has been shown to reduce body weight in clozapine patients[27]. Structured cognitive-behavioural therapy (CBT) may also be useful[26], especially in those with binge eating symptoms[28]. Of the many pharmacological treatments which have been investigated to reverse antipsychotic-induced weight gain (*Table 5.3.4*), metformin is the most widely studied and supported[29, 30]. *Table 5.3.4* outlines the pharmacological approaches used to reduce clozapine-induced weight gain.

Table 5.3.4: Pharmacological approaches to clozapine-induced weight gain[31]

Drug (type of study)	No of patients	Trial duration	Change in body weight	Comment
Aripiprazole[32] (RCT)	207	RCT 16 weeks with 12 week open extension	-2.53 kg in the aripiprazole arm vs. -0.38 kg in the placebo arm ($p<0.001$). The improvement was maintained during the open extension	BMI and waist circumference also improved. No significant difference in PANSS between groups (p=0.370)
Atomoxetine[33] (RCT)	37	24 weeks	A trend to weight loss was seen in both atomoxetine and placebo arms. No significant difference noted	The authors conclude that atomoxetine is not effective for weight loss in clozapine patients
Metformin[34] (RCT)	40 on clozapine	12 weeks	- 3.2kg metformin alone - 4.7kg metformin + lifestyle interventions	Metformin alone or in combination with lifestyle interventions demonstrated efficacy. Clozapine was one of four atypical antipsychotics included in the study
Meta-analysis[35]	One out of 6 RCTs included patients on clozapine	12–16 weeks	Average weight reduction was 3.16kg, BMI reduction 1.21kg/m2, waist circumference -1.99cm	Meta-analysis of 6 RCTs investigating the use of metformin to reduce the metabolic impact of atypical antipsychotics
Modafinil[36] (RCT)	35	8 weeks	Weight and BMI improved in the modafinil arm, but not significantly greater than placebo (p=0.07)	The study may have been underpowered to detect a significant improvement
Orlistat[37,38] (RCT followed by an open labelled study)	63 RCT 44 Open label	16-week RCT followed by 16-week	Only males showed an improvement over placebo (– 2.36 kgs vs. 0.62kg, P=0.011)	There was no formal calorie-controlled diet followed during the trials. The open label extension study showed no

Table 5.3.4: Pharmacological approaches to clozapine-induced weight gain *continued*

Drug (type of study)	No of patients	Trial duration	Change in body weight	Comment
Orlistat[37,38] *continued*		open labelled study		additional benefits to those seen with the RCT
Quetiapine[39] (Retrospective study)	65	10 months	Mean change of -1.85kg after the first month of combination	Clozapine dose reduced by 25% when quetiapine added Quetiapine commonly causes sedation and hypotension which may be accentuated with clozapine
Sibutramine[40] (RCT)	21	12 weeks	No significant changes in weight or BMI reported	The sample size may have been too small to show a difference. No longer widely available Note: Sibutramine was withdrawn from the European and US market in 2010 over fears of an increased risk of cardiovascular events[41]

In addition to the medication listed in *Table 5.3.4*, there are single case reports of memantine[42], topiramate[43] and acetazolamide[44] reducing clozapine-induced weight gain.

Summary

- Although all antipsychotics have been shown to cause weight gain, clozapine and olanzapine are consistently associated with the greatest increases.
- Similar to other antipsychotics, the most rapid period of weight gain with clozapine is in the first few months of treatment.
- While the weight gain from other antipsychotics generally plateaus within a year, it may take up to four years for weight to stabilise for those on clozapine.
- One-fifth of all patients receiving clozapine may gain 10% of their baseline body weight.
- The mechanisms behind weight gain with clozapine are multifactorial and probably involve a combination of receptor, hormonal and genetic influences.
- All patients should be counselled about the risks of weight gain with clozapine and how to maintain a healthy diet and active lifestyle, both before starting and regularly throughout treatment.

- Those with a high BMI or waist circumference should be encouraged to engage in a calorie controlled diet and a structured physical health exercise programme.
- The addition of aripiprazole or metformin may also help reduce weight in individuals receiving clozapine. Metformin is considered the drug of choice to prevent and treat clozapine-induced weight gain.

Further reading and resources

Haddad P. Weight changes with atypical antipsychotics in the treatment of schizophrenia. *J Psychopharmacol* 2005; **19(Suppl):** 16–27

Lett T, Wallace T, Chowdhury N, Tiwari A, Kennedy J, Muller D. Pharmacogenetics of antipsychotic-induced weight gain. Review and clinical implications. *Mol Psychiatry* 2012; **17:** 242–66

www.qrisk.org – The Q-risk 2012 calculator. Calculates the 10 year risk of myocardial infarction or strokes. Developed for the National Health Service in the UK

References

1. World Health Organisation. *Overweight and Obesity. Fact sheet No 311*. May 2012. Geneva; World Health Organisation: 2012. Available at: www.who.int
2. National Collaborating Centre for Primary Care and the Centre for Public Health Excellence. *Obesity: the prevention, identification, assessment and management of overweight and obesity adults and children. (NICE Clinical Guideline CG43)*. National Institute for Health and Clinical Excellence, 2006
3. Centre for Disease control and prevention. *Calculation of BMI*. Available at: www.cdc.gov. (assessed January 2013)
4. Haddad P. Weight changes with atypical antipsychotics in the treatment of schizophrenia. *J Psychopharmacol* 2005; **19(Suppl):** 16–27
5. Taylor D, McAskill R. Atypical antipsychotics and weight gain — a systematic review. *Acta Psychiatr Scand* 2000; **101:** 416–32
6. Allison D, Mentore J, Heo M, Chandler L, Cappelleri J, Infante M, et al. Antipsychotic-induced weight gain: A comprehensive research synthesis. *Am J Psychiatry* 1999; **156:** 1686–96
7. Rummel-Kluge C, Komossa K, Schwarz S, Hunger H, Schmid F, Asenjo C, et al. Head-to-head comparisons of metabolic side effects of second generation antipsychotics in the treatment of schizophrenia: a systematic review and meta-analysis. *Schizophr Res* 2010; **123:** 225–33
8. Wetterling T. Bodyweight gain with atypical antipsychotics: A comparative review. *Drug Safety* 2001; **24:** 59–73
9. Henderson D, Cagliero E, Gray C, Nasrallah R, Hayden D, Schoenfeld D, et al. Clozapine, diabetes mellitus, weight gain, and lipid abnormalities: a five-year naturalistic study. *Am J Psychiatry* 2000; **157:** 975–81
10. Henderson D, Nguyen D, Copeland P, Hayden D, Borba C, Louie P, et al. Clozapine, diabetes mellitus, hyperlipidaemia, and cardiovascular risks and mortality: results of a 10-year naturalistic study. *J Clin Psychiatry* 2005; **66:** 1116–21
11. Haro J, Edgell E, Jones P, Alonso J, Gavart S, Gregor K, et al, The European schizophrenia outpatient health

outcomes (SOHO) study: rationale, methods and recruitment. *Acta Psychiatr Scand* 2003; **107:** 222–32

12. Safferman A, Lieberman J, Kane J, Szymanski S, KinonB. Update on the clinical efficacy and side effects of clozapine. *Schizophr Bull* 1991; **17:** 247–61
13. Simon V, van Winkel R, De Hert M. Are weight gain and metabolic side effects of atypical antipsychotics dose dependent? A literature review. *J Clin Psychiatry* 2009; **70:** 1041–50
14. Stahl S, Mignon L, Meyer J. Which comes first: atypical antipsychotic treatment or cardiometabolic risk? *Acta Psychiatr Scand* 2009; **119:** 171–9
15. Meltzer H. Illumining the molecular basis for some antipsychotic drug-induced metabolic burden. *Proc Natl Acad Sci U S A* 2007; **104:** 3019–20
16. Hägg S, Söderberg S, Ahrén B, Olsson T, Mjörndal T. Leptin concentrations are increased in subjects treated with clozapine or conventional antipsychotics. *J Clin Psychiatry* 2001; **62:** 843–8
17. Baptista T, Beaulieu S. Are leptin and cytokines involved in body weight gain during treatment with antipsychotic drugs? *Can J Psychiatry* 2002; **47:** 742–9
18. Theisen F, Gebhardt S, Haberhausen M, Heinzel-Gutenbrunner M, Wehmeier P, Krieg J, et al. Clozapine-induced weight gain: a study in monozygotic twins and same-sex sib pairs. *Psychiatr Genet* 2005; **15:** 285–9
19. Lett T, Wallace T, Chowdhury N, Tiwari A, Kennedy J, Muller D. Pharmacogenetics of antipsychotic-induced weight gain. Review and clinical implications. *Mol Psychiatry* 2012; **17:** 242–66
20. Bai Y, Lin CC, Chen JY, Lin CYn Su TP, Ph PC. Association of initial antipsychotic response to clozapine and long-term weight gain. *Am J Psychiatry* 2006; **163:** 1276–9
21. Meltzer H, Perry E, Jayathilake K. Clozapine-induced weight gain predicts improvement in psychopathology. *Schizophr Res* 2002; **59:** 19–27
22. Signore A, Zhang F, Weng Z, Gao Y, Chen J. Leptin neuroprotection in the CNS: mechanisms and therapeutic potentials. *J Neurochem* 2008; **106:** 1977–90
23. Wirshing D, Smith R, Erickson Z, Mena S, Wirshing W. A wellness class for inpatients with psychotic disorders. *J Psychiatr Practice* 2006; **12:** 24–9
24. Alvarez-Jimenez M, Gonzalez-Blanch C, Vazquez-Barquero J, Perez-Iglesias R, Martínez-García O, Pérez-Pardal T, et al. Attenuation of antipsychotic-induced weight gain with early behavioural intervention in drug-naive first-episode psychosis patients: A randomized controlled trial. *J Clin Psychiatry* 2006; **67:** 1253–60
25. Mauri M, Castrogiovanni S, Simoncini M, Iovieno N, Miniati M, Rossi A, et al. Effects of an educational intervention on weight gain in patients treated with antipsychotics. *J Clin Psychopharmacol* 2006; **26:** 462–6
26. Faulkner G, Cohn T, Remington G. Interventions to reduce weight gain in schizophrenia. Cochrane Database of Systematic Reviews 2007, Issue 1. Art. No.: CD005148. DOI: 10.1002/14651858. CD005148.pub2.
27. Wu M, Wang C, Bai Y, Huang C, Lee S. Outcomes of obese, clozapine-treated inpatients with schizophrenia placed on a six-month diet and physical activity programme. *Psychiatr Serv* 2007; **58:** 544–50
28. Khazaal Y, Fresard E, Rabia S, Chatton A, Rothen S, Pomini V et al. Cognitive behavioural therapy for weight gain associated with antipsychotic drugs. *Schizophr Res* 2007; **91:** 169–77
29. De Hert M, Dekker J, Wood D, Kahl K, Holt R, Möller HJ. Cardiovascular disease and diabetes in people

with severe mental illness position statement from the European Psychiatric Association (EPA), supported by the European Association for the Study of Diabetes (EASD) and the European Society of Cardiology (ESC). *Eur Psychiatry* 2009; **24:** 412–24

30. Taylor D, Paton C, Kapur S. *The Maudsley Prescribing Guidelines.* 11th edn: Oxford: Wiley-Blackwell: 2012

31. Baptista T, ElFakih Y, Uzcategui E, Sandia I, Talamo E, de Baptista E, et al. Pharmacological management of atypical antipsychotic-induced weight gain. *CNS Drugs* 2008; **22:** 477–95

32. Fleischhacker W, Heikkinen M, Olié J-P, Landsberg W, Dewaele P, McQuade R, et al. Effects of adjunctive treatment with aripiprazole on body weight and clinical efficacy in schizophrenia patients treated with clozapine: a randomized, double-blind, placebo-controlled trial. *Int J Neuropsychopharmacol* 2010; **13:** 1115–25

33. Ball M, Warren K, Feldman S, McMahon R, Kelly R, Buchanan R. Placebo-controlled trial of atomoxetine for weight reduction in people with schizophrenia treated with clozapine or olanzapine. *Clin Schizophr Rel Psychoses* 2011; **5:** 17–25

34. Wu R, Zhao J, Jin H, Shao P, Fang M, Guo X, et al. Lifestyle intervention and metformin for treatment of antipsychotic-induced weight gain. *J Am Med Assoc* 2008; **299:** 185–93

35. Ehret M, Goethe J, Lanosa M, Coleman C. The effect of metformin on anthropometrics and insulin resistance in patients receiving atypical antipsychotics agents: A meta-analysis. *J Clin Psychiatry* 2010; **71:** 1286–92

36. Henderson D, Freudenreich O, Bora C, Wang X, Copeland P, Macklin E, et al. Effects of modafinil on weight, glucose and lipid metabolism in clozapine-treated patients with schizophrenia. *Schizophr Res* 2011; **130:** 53–6

37. Joffe G, Takala P, Tchoukhine E, Hakko H, Raidma M, Putkonen H, et al. Orlistat in clozapine or olanzapine treated patients with overweight or obesity: a 16-week randomized, double-blind, placebo-controlled trial. *J Clin Psychiatry* 2008; **69:** 706–11

38. Tchoukhine E, Takala P, Hakko H, Raidma M, Putkonen H, Räsänen P, et al. Orlistat in clozapine or olanzapine treated patients with overweight or obesity: A 16-week open-label extension phase and both phases of a randomized controlled trial. *J Clin Psychiatry* 2011; **72:** 326–30

39. Reinstein MJ, Sirotovskaya LA, Jones LE, Mohan S, Chasanov MA. Effect of clozapine-quetiapine combination therapy on weight and glycaemic control: preliminary findings. *Clin Drug Invest* 1999; **18:** 99–104

40. Henderson D, Fan X, Copeland P, Borba C, Daley T, Nguyen D, et al. A double-blind, placebo-controlled trial of sibutramine for clozapine associated weight gain. *Acta Psychiatr Scand* 2007; **115:** 101–5

41. Martindale: The Complete Drug Reference. [online] London: Pharmaceutical Press. Available at: www.medicinescomplete.com (accessed 7 January 2013)

42. Schaefer M, Leopold K, Hinzpeter A, Heinz A, Krebs M. Memantine-associated reversal of clozapine-induced weight gain. *Pharmacopsychiatry* 2007; **40:** 149–51

43. Dursun S, Devarajan S. Clozapine weight gain, plus topiramate weight loss. *Can J Psychiatry* 2000; **45:** 198

44. Schneiderhan M, Marvin R. Is acetazolamide similar to topiramate for reversal of antipsychotic-induced weight gain? *Am J Therapeutics* 2007; **14:** 581–4

5.4: Dyslipidaemia and metabolic syndrome

Cardiovascular disease (CVD) is the number one cause of death globally[1] and dyslipidaemia is one of the major modifiable risk factors for developing CVD (along with smoking and high blood pressure)[2]. As the concentration of total cholesterol increases so does the risk of CVD[3]. Current recommendations suggest that all adults over the age of 40 years should have their cholesterol levels measured as part of a CVD prevention programme[2,3]. Any individual who presents with a 20% or greater risk of having a cardiovascular event in the next 10 years should be actively treated with a lipid lowering drug such as a statin[3]. For those with diabetes more aggressive treatment is recommended[3]. Effective lipid control has a dramatic effect on outcome. In an early meta-analysis of statin trials, a 10% reduction in low-density lipoprotein cholesterol (LDL-C) was shown to reduce the risk of CVD by 25% after five years[4].

Schizophrenia and dyslipidaemia

People with serious mental illnesses such as schizophrenia have a 2–3-fold increased mortality compared with the general population and the commonest cause of natural death is from CVD (the median standard mortality rate for CVD in schizophrenia is 1.79, 90% quantiles 1.11–3.60)[5]. While there are likely to be many causes for this increased risk (e.g. increased smoking rates, obesity, diabetes and poor self-care), dyslipidaemia is a significant factor which is often neglected and undertreated. Evidence from the Clinical Antipsychotic Trials of Intervention Effectiveness (CATIE) reported that 88% (n=1445) of those with dyslipidaemia received no treatment[5]. Further literature from the US reports that less than 10% of those prescribed a second generation antipsychotic have a baseline lipid measurement (n=55,436)[7]. A UK-wide audit of metabolic screening in outpatients prescribed antipsychotics reported a lipid screen in just 28% of patients[7]. Extrapolating from population estimates the authors concluded that for every case of dyslipidaemia identified, seven were missed[8].

Clozapine and dyslipidaemia

The association between antipsychotics and dyslipidaemia has been less well studied than the incidence of diabetes and weight gain. Both first generation and second generation antipsychotics have been shown to cause dyslipidaemia[10], but the extent of the effect varies greatly between antipsychotics. Clozapine, olanzapine and quetiapine appear to cause the most profound elevations in cholesterol, while aripiprazole and ziprasidone have the least effect[10, 11]. While this mirrors the trend seen with antipsychotic-induced weight gain, even in the absence of weight gain antipsychotics can cause dyslipdaemia[12].

Short-term RCTs (14 weeks or less) have shown that clozapine increases total cholesterol and triglyceride levels[11, 13, 14]. Over a longer period (up to 10 years follow-up), triglyceride elevation seen with clozapine remains consistently high, but the total cholesterol changes are often small and not significant[15, 16]. Elevated triglycerides without changes in total cholesterol still increases CVD risk and may reflect smaller, denser, triglyceride-rich LDL cholesterol, which is less readily cleared by normal pathways[3]. The mean increase of triglycerides for clozapine at eight weeks has been shown to be 0.35mmol/L[14], which increases to 1.86mmol/L over five years[17]. For most people this would represent a near doubling of their triglyceride level with long-term treatment. Although there appears to be a relationship between clozapine plasma levels and triglyceride levels, it is unclear how significant this is[17, 18]. The mechanism behind clozapine-induced dyslipidaemia is not well understood. There is a clear link between weight gain, insulin resistance and dyslipidaemia, and it is likely that many of the mechanisms discussed in other chapters are relevant to dyslipidaemia. Second generation antipsychotics have been shown to increase lipogenesis, reduce lipolysis and enhance the antilipolytic effects of insulin[19] — all of which causes an increase in lipids in adipose tissue. Large-scale population studies are beginning to unravel the genetic influences associated with dyslipidaemia[20] and hopefully with further research a clearer mechanism, which can be directly influenced, will become apparent. Specific risk factors for clozapine-related dyslipidaemia are also unclear. Certainly familial hypercholesterolaemia would be a concern when starting clozapine and thus should be actively treated.

Treatment for clozapine-induced dyslipidaemia

Improving the rates of lipid monitoring for all people on antipsychotics will very probably reduce mortality in schizophrenia through reducing the risk of CVDs. Monitoring should begin with a baseline full lipid profile and investigating for familial hypercholesterolaemia. A fasting sample (a fast of 9–12 hours) gives more accurate results for LDL cholesterol, but even a non-fasting sample is helpful. As there is a natural variation in lipid levels from day to day (total cholesterol can vary by 10%), repeat measurements should be considered to give a complete picture[9]. Treatment is usually targeted for those who have underlying CVD risk factors (smoking, hypertension, diabetes, etc) and an LDL-C greater than 2mmol/L. Blood testing for lipids should be repeated after the first and third months of clozapine treatment, then regularly every six months on long-term treatment.

Advice on a healthy diet and active lifestyle should be given at every opportunity for those on clozapine. People with mild to moderately elevated cholesterol levels may be able to reach target levels by altering their diet (e.g. eating lean meat, fish and reducing saturated fat intake)[5] and improving physical activity. Dietary changes and physical activity programmes have been shown to be effective in reducing clozapine-induced triglyceride changes over six months[21].

For others, active treatment with a statin is recommended. Statins have been shown to be effective in reducing both triglyceride and total cholesterol levels in those prescribed clozapine[22]. Statins are generally well tolerated but can rarely cause rhabdomyolyosis (incidence of 0.01%)[5] and liver dysfunction. A baseline creatinine kinase and liver function tests are recommended, which are repeated if any symptoms emerge. Other drugs (e.g. fibrates) are occasionally used, following specialist advice, either in combination with a statin if target lipids levels are not achieved or when statins are poorly tolerated.

Other approaches to reduce clozapine-induced dyslipidaemia include omega-3 supplementation (triglycerides reduce but LDL-C may increase)[23], orlistat[24] and augmenting clozapine with aripiprazole[25].

Metabolic syndrome and clozapine

Metabolic syndrome is a constellation of other symptoms, which, when occurring together, synergistically increase the risk and mortality from CVD and type 2 diabetes[26]. Many definitions have been proposed and the most recent international consensus[27] suggests that metabolic syndrome is established if any three of the following five criteria are present:

- Elevated waist circumference (≥94 cm men, ≥80cm women, of European descent)
- Raised triglycerides (≥1.7mmol/L or ≥150mg/dL) or drug treatment for dyslipidaemia
- Reduced HDL cholesterol (≤1.03mmol/L or ≤40mg/dL) or drug treatment for dyslipidaemia
- Elevated blood pressure (systolic ≥130mmHg, diastolic ≥ 85mmHg) or a history of hypertension or drug treatment for hypertension
- Elevated fasting glucose (≥5.6 mmol/L or ≥100mg/dL) or drug treatment for hyperglycaemia.

The prevalence of metabolic syndrome reported in people with schizophrenia varies greatly, depending on the definition used and population demographics (3.9–68% have been reported)[28]. Metabolic syndrome appears more likely with the second generation antipsychotics compared with first generation, and clozapine and olanzapine have the highest rates[28]. Over half of people (54%) receiving clozapine are reported to have metabolic syndrome[29].

Treatment of metabolic syndrome is identical to treating the individual components. Regular monitoring and pre-screening for risk factors is essential, followed up with advice on maintaining a healthy diet and lifestyle. Appropriate drug therapy should be introduced at an early stage in an attempt to reduce the extensive risks associated with CVD and diabetes.

Table 5.4.1: Lipid targets in those with established CVD, diabetes, or people with a 20% or greater risk of CVD over 10 years[2,3,9]

The main lipids in serum	Target recommendations to reduce CVD risk	Comments
High-density lipoprotein cholesterol (HDL-C)	No specific target although risk may be greater with levels <1.0mmol/l in men or <1.2mmol/L in women	Inverse association with CVD. High levels are protective, low levels are a risk factor. Can usually be measured in a non-fasting state
Low-density lipoprotein cholesterol (LDL-C)	Less than 2.0mmol/l or a 30% reduction in LDL-C	80% of total cholesterol in serum is contained in LDL-C. The preferred target for cholesterol lowering. Best measured in a fasting state
Triglycerides	No specific target although >1.7 mmol/L is considered to be hypertriglyceridaemia	Hypertriglyceridaemia increases CVD risk probably by causing an increase in triglyceride-rich lipoproteins. Best measured in a fasting state
Total cholesterol (TC)	Less than 4.0mmol/l or a 25% reduction in total cholesterol	Can usually be measured in a non-fasting state

Summary

- Dyslipidaemia is one of the major modifiable risk factors for developing coronary vascular diseases.
- Clozapine appears to have a significant effect on triglyceride levels which can double with long-term therapy.
- All people prescribed clozapine should have a baseline lipid profile (ideally a fasting sample), which should be repeated after the first and third months of treatment.
- Lipid profile monitoring should be repeated every six months for those on long-term treatment.
- People with mild to moderately elevated cholesterol levels may be able to reach target levels by altering their diet and improving physical activity.
- For others, a statin is recommended and generally well tolerated.
- Over half of all people receiving clozapine may have metabolic syndrome.

Further reading and resources

Young I. Lipids for psychiatrists: an overview. *J Psychopharmacol* 2005; **19(suppl):** 66–75

Papanastasiou E. The prevalence and mechanisms of metabolic syndrome in schizophrenia: a review. *Therapeut Adv Psychopharmacol* 2012; **0:** 1–19

www.qrisk.org: The Q-risk 2012 calculator. Calculates the 10-year risk of myocardial infarction or strokes. Developed for the National Health Service in the UK

References

1. World Health Organization. Cardiovascular Diseases. Factsheet No 317. September 2012. Geneva; available at: www.who.int (accessed January 2013)
2. National Collaborating Centre for Primary Care and Royal College of General Practitioners. *Clinical Guidelines and Evidence Review for Lipid Modification: cardiovascular risk assessment and the primary and secondary prevention of cardiovascular disease. (NICE Guidelines CG67)*. National Institute for Health and Clinical Excellence May 2008
3. Joint British Societies. Joint British Societies' guidelines on prevention of cardiovascular disease in clinical practice. *Heart* 2005; **91(Suppl V):** 1–52
4. Law M, Wald N, Thompson S. By how much and how quickly does reduction in serum cholesterol concentration lower risk of ischaemic heart disease? *Br Med J* 1994; **308:** 367–72
5. De Hert M, Dekker J, Wood D, Kahl K, Holt R, Möller HJ. Cardiovascular disease and diabetes in people with severe mental illness position statement from the European Psychiatric Association (EPA), supported by the European Association for the Study of Diabetes (EASD) and the European Society of Cardiology (ESC). *Eur Psychiatry* 2009; **24:** 412–24
6. Nasrallah H, Meyer J, Goff D, McEvoy J, Davis S, Stroup T, et al. Low rates of treatment for hypertension, dyslipidemia and diabetes in schizophrenia: data from the CATIE schizophrenia trial sample at baseline. *Schizophr Res* 2006; **86:** 15–22
7. Morrato E, Newcomer J, Allen R, Valuck R. Prevalence of baseline serum glucose and lipid testing in users of second-generation antipsychotic drugs: a retrospective, population-based study of Medicaid claims data. *J Clin Psychiatry* 2008; **69:** 316–22
8. Barnes T, Paton C, Cavanagh M, Hancock E, Taylor D. A UK audit of screening for the metabolic side-effects of antipsychotics in community patients. *Schizophr Bull* 2007; **33:** 1397–1403
9. Young I. Lipids for psychiatrists — an overview. *J Psychopharmacol* 2005; **19(suppl):** 66–75
10. Koro C, Fedder D, L'Italien G, Weiss S, Magder L, Kreyenbuhl J, et al. An assessment of the independent effects of olanzapine and risperidone exposure on the risk of hyperlipidemia in schizophrenic patients. *Arch General Psychiatry* 2002; **59:** 1021–6
11. Rummel-Kluge C, Komossa K, Schwarz S, Hunger H, Schmid F, Asenjo C, et al. Head-to-head comparisons of metabolic side-effects of second generation antipsychotics in the treatment of schizophrenia: a systematic review and meta-analysis. *Schizophr Res* 2010; **123:** 225–33
12. Stahl S, Mignon L, Meyer J. Which comes first: atypical antipsychotic treatment or cardiometabolic risk? *Acta Psychiatr Scand* 2009; **119:** 171–9
13. Lindenmayer J, Czobor P, Volavka J, Citrome L, Sheitman B, McEnvoy J, et al. Changes in glucose and cholesterol levels in patients with schizophrenia and treated with typical or atypical antipsychotics. *Am J Psychiatry* 2003; **160:** 290–6
14. Wu R, Zhao J, Liu Z, Zhai J, Guo X, Guo, W, et al. Effects of typical and atypical antipsychotics on glucose–insulin homeostasis and lipid metabolism in first-episode schizophrenia. *Psychopharmacol* 2006; **186:** 572–8
15. Henderson D, Nguyen D, Copeland P, Hayden D, Borba C, Louie P, et al. Clozapine, diabetes mellitus, hyperlipidaemia, and cardiovascular risks and mortality: results of a 10-year naturalistic study. *J Clin Psychiatry* 2005; **66:** 1116–21

16. Gaulin B, Markowita J, Caley C, Nesbitt L, Dufresne R. Clozapine-associated elevation in serum triglycerides. *Am J Psychiatry* 1999; **156:** 1270–2
17. Henderson D, Cagliero E, Gray C, Nasrallah R, Hayden D, Schoenfeld D, et al. Clozapine, diabetes mellitus, weight gain, and lipid abnormalities: a five-year naturalistic study. *Am J Psychiatry* 2000; **157:** 975–81
18. Simon V, van Winkel R, De Hert M. Are weight gain and metabolic side effects of atypical antipsychotics dose dependent? A literature review. *J Clin Psychiatry* 2009; **70:** 1041–50
19. Chaggar P, Shaw S, Williams S. Effect of antipsychotic medications on glucose and lipid levels. *J Clin Pharmacol* 2011; **51:** 631–8
20. Teslovich T, Musunuru K, Smith A, Edmondson A, Stylianou I, Koseki M. Biological, clinical and population relevance of 95 loci for blood lipids. *Nature* 2010; **466:** 707–13
21. Wu M, Wang C, Bai Y, Huang C, Lee S. Outcomes of obese, clozapine-treated inpatients with schizophrenia placed on a six-month diet and physical activity programme. *Psychiatr Serv* 2007; **58:** 544–50
22. Landry P, Dimitri E, Tessier S, Légaré N. Efficacy of lipid-lowering medications in patients treated with clozapine. *J Clin Psychopharmacol* 2008; **28:** 348–9
23. Caniato R, Alvarenga M, Garcia-Alcaraz M. Effect of omega-3 fatty acids on the lipid profile of patients taking clozapine. *Aust N Z J Psychiatry* 2006; **40:** 691–7
24. Tchoukhine E, Takala P, Hakko H, Raidma M, Putkonen H, Räsänen P, et al. Orlistat in clozapine-or olanzapine-treated patients with overweight or obesity: A 16-week open-label extension phase and both phases of a randomized controlled trial. *J Clinical Psychiatry* 2011; **72:** 326–30
25. Fleischhacker W, Heikkinen M, Olié J-P, Landsberg W, Dewaele P, McQuade R, et al. Effects of adjunctive treatment with aripiprazole on body weight and clinical efficacy in schizophrenia patients treated with clozapine: a randomized, double-blind, placebo-controlled trial. *Int J Neuropsychopharmacol* 2010; **13:** 1115–25
26. Eckel, R, Grundy S, Zimmet P. The metabolic syndrome. *Lancet* 2005; **365:** 1415–28
27. Alberti K, Eckel R, Grundy S, Zimmet P, Cleeman J, Donato K, et al. Harmonizing the metabolic syndrome. *Circulation* 2009; **120:** 1640–5
28. Papanastasiou E. The prevalence and mechanisms of metabolic syndrome in schizophrenia: a review. *Ther Adv Psychopharmacol* 2012; **0:** 1–19
29. Lamberti J, Olson D, Crilly J, Olivares T, Williams G, Tu X, et al. Prevalence of the metabolic syndrome among patients receiving clozapine. *Am J Psychiatry* 2006; **163:** 1273–6

5.5: Gastrointestinal hypomotility and constipation

Clozapine-induced gastrointestinal hypomotility (CIGH) is common, under-investigated and associated with rare, but rapidly fatal consequences. Clozapine can affect the entire gastrointestinal system ranging from swallowing difficulties to rectal bleeding. Constipation is reported in 14–60% of clozapine users[1] and, although this is often benign, there have been many case reports of deaths associated with: aspiration of vomit secondary to bowel obstruction[2, 3], toxic megacolon[4], necrotising colitis[5, 6], colonic perforation, abdominal compartment syndrome[7] and bowel infarction[8] (*Table 5.5.1*). Other causes of death or life-threatening illness where severe CIGH was a likely cause includes septic shock, organ failure, pneumonia and cardiac abmormalities[1]. The prevalence of life-threatening CIGH has been estimated as three cases per 1000 patients exposed to clozapine[1].

As of April 2013, the Medicines and Healthcare products Regulatory Authority (MHRA) in the UK had received 5061 reports of gastrointestinal adverse reactions suspected of being associated with clozapine, of which 82 were fatal. This compares with just five fatalities from blood disorders over the same time period[9]. National alerts on CIGH have been issued by the UK, New Zealand and Canadian medicines authorities[10–12].

Of particular concern is the sudden and rapid deterioration of health reported in some of these fatalities. In many cases, the first symptoms were only reported a few hours or days before death[1, 8]. This may be explained by the observation that those with schizophrenia have a reduced pain sensitivity[13], and many will also be receiving analgesics, antidepressants or anticonvulsants which can further suppress pain.

There appear to be three main mechanisms associated with severe or life-threatening consequences of CIGH[1]:

- Untreated bowel obstruction leads to distension, necrosis, perforation or sepsis
- Aspiration from faecal vomiting
- Faecal stasis leading to infection.

Symptoms reported in life-threatening cases of CIGH include: constipation, abdominal pain or cramp, fever, nausea, diarrhoea (overflow), distended abdomen, pneumonia or drowsiness[1, 14] . However, in some cases the onset is so rapid that few specific symptoms are reported.

Risk factors for developing complications include a higher dose of clozapine or a higher plasma level in conjunction with interacting drugs or stopping smoking, co-prescribing of other drugs which commonly cause constipation (other anticholinergics, opiates, anti-diarrhoea medication), a low-fibre diet, dehydration (which can be exacerbated by clozapine-induced hypersalivation), obesity, poor bowel function and a lack of exercise[1,14]. Although constipation can occur at any time during clozapine treatment, the first four months are associated with a slightly higher risk of complications (36% of life-threatening cases occurred within the first four months in one study)[1].

Pathophysiology of CIGH

The mechanism behind CIGH is generally considered to be because of clozapine's potent antagonism at acetylcholine receptors. Acetylcholine stimulates muscarinic receptors on intestinal smooth muscle cells increasing gut motility and tone. Drugs such as clozapine, which are anticholinergic, oppose these affects and therefore commonly cause constipation. However, clozapine is associated with more gastrointestinal hypomotility than other equally anticholinergic agents, so antagonism of serotonin receptors may also play a role[1,7].

Clozapine antagonises serotonin 5-HT_2, 5-HT_3, 5-HT_6 and 5-HT_7 receptors. Up to 95% of the body's serotonin receptors are found in the gastrointestinal tract and 5-HT_3 antagonism is associated with reduced motility and constipation[7]. Other 5-HT_3 antagonists in medical use include ondansetron and granisetron (used as antiemetics in chemotherapy), and they also commonly cause constipation.

Treatment of CIGH

There are no clinical studies published examining the specific treatment of CIGH. Treatment should focus on preventing symptoms occurring, active screening throughout treatment and the assertive use of laxatives[1]. Preventing symptoms includes screening for any underlying bowel problems before starting clozapine, advising on the risks of constipation, ensuring adequate fibre, fluid and exercise. Referring to a dietician at an early stage may also be useful. Although increasing dietary fibre can increase stool weight and decrease gut transit time, adequate fluid must be ensured to avoid obstruction. Adults should aim to consume 18–30g per day of fibre, drink 6–8 medium glasses of fluid a day, and do at least 150 minutes of physical activity a week[14].

Clozapine-induced constipation can rapidly become fatal so clinicians should have a low threshold for starting laxatives. In chronic constipation, stopping any medication which is contributing and reducing the clozapine dose, are also important to consider.

There is no clear evidence indicating which laxatives are superior in CIGH. In general, laxatives are divided into four groups: bulk forming, stimulant, osmotic and faecal softeners. Many laxatives have complex modes of action across different groups and choice is often guided by previous response, tolerability and required speed of action. The following is a brief guide to the different laxatives and readers are reminded to seek specialist advice.

Table 5.5.1: Published cases of deaths associated with CIGH

Author	Age/ sex	Daily dose of clozapine at the time of death	Duration of clozapine treatment	Concurrent contributing medication	Onset of symptoms	Recorded cause of death
Drew et al, 1997[3]	49 male	500mg	2 years	Nil of note	A few hours	Inhalation of faeculant vomitus
Eronen et al, 2003[4]	36 male	500mg	Unknown	Loperamide 6mg in one day	16 hours	Toxic megacolon
Flanagan et al, 2011[15]	41 male	750mg	6 years	Nil of note	One day	Aspiration complicating severe, constipation
Hayes at al, 1995[2]	29 male	400mg	36 days	Not recorded	Not recorded	Aspiration of vomitus
Hibbard et al, 2009[7]	61 male	600mg	7 years	Procyclidine 5mg BD Oxybutynin 5mg BD	3 days (intermittent constipation preceding 12 years)	Aspiration of feculent vomitus
Hibbard et al, 2009[7]	63 male	400mg	16 days	Nil of note	A few days	Abdominal compartment syndrome
Levin et al, 2002[6]	43 male	750mg	Six years	Nil of note	Few hours	Septic shock
Seller et al, 2006[16]	43 male	700mg	10 years	Nil of note	Not recorded	Cardiac arrest in surgery following a necrotic and ischaemic bowel
Seller et al, 2006[16]	23 male	400mg	Not recorded	Not recorded	3 days	Bowel perforation
Seller et al, 2006[16]	56 male	400mg	15 years	Not recorded	Chronic constipation noted	Unclear
Shammi et al, 1997[5]	36 male	600mg	4 months	Benztropine 2mg daily	1 day (constipation was an ongoing problem)	Necrotising colitis
Townsend, 2006[8]	20 male	900mg	One year	Not recorded	2 days	Infarction of the bowel
Fayad et al, 2012[19]	65 male	100mg	Nine days	Olanzapine	Not recorded	Complication of adynamic ileus

Bulk forming laxatives (e.g. ispaghula husks or methylcellulose)

These relieve constipation by increasing faecal mass which stimulates peristalsis. They may be of value in those with small hard stools but can take many days to work. The patient must be advised to have an adequate fluid intake and should avoid taking them last thing at night. While they are suitable for long-term use, they are contraindicated in obstruction, colonic atony and faecal impaction[17, 18], which clozapine patients may be particularly prone to. The treatment of uncomplicated constipation usually starts with introducing a bulk forming laxative, but as CIGH can be quickly life-threatening the clinician should not hesitate to prescribe faster-acting laxatives.

Osmotic laxatives (e.g. lactulose, macrogols, phosphate and sodium citrate enemas)

These act by increasing the amount of fluid in the large bowel. As with bulk forming laxatives, an adequate fluid intake is important to prevent the potential dehydrating effects which can exacerbate constipation. A high dose of macrogol oral powders can be used to treat faecal impaction and the enemas can prove useful in removing hard impacted stools[17,18].

Stimulant laxatives (e.g. senna, bisacodyl and glycerol suppositories)

These work by stimulating rectal or colonic nerves causing increased peristalsis. The onset of effect is usually rapid (around 12 hours with the oral preparations) and they can be useful when bulk forming and osmotic laxatives have proved ineffective, or when a rapid effect is required[17, 18]. Stimulant laxatives are often required for the effective treatment of clozapine-related constipation. They should not be withheld, delayed or prematurely withdrawn.

Faecal softeners (e.g. arachis oil enemas)

These lubricate and soften impacted faeces. They take many hours to work, so are usually used overnight and are followed by a potent osmotic enema such as a phosphate enema.

All healthcare professionals should actively enquire about symptoms of CIGH and have a low threshold for treatment and investigation. While this can prove challenging in an acute, mentally unwell patient, the potential consequences can be sudden and life-threatening.

Figure 5.5.1 provides a suggested algorithm for preventing and treating CIGH.

Figure 5.5.1: Algorithm for treating CIGH

Before starting clozapine Advise on adequate fibre, fluid and exercise. Investigate underlying bowel function and frequency of motions. Warn patients on the risks associated with constipation and the importance of seeking medical advice Review the need for any concurrent medication which can cause constipation (e.g. anticholinergics, opiates and anti-motility medication)
During clozapine treatment Regularly enquire about bowel habits and frequency. Reinforce the advice regarding adequate fibre in the diet, fluid intake and exercise
CIGH suspected Choice of laxative is often guided by previous response, tolerability and required speed of action. In uncomplicated cases, bulk forming laxatives such as ispaghula husks or methylcellulose may be appropriate. In cases of sudden onset and deteriorating physical health, expert advice should immediately be sought and clinicians should begin potent stimulant or osmotic laxatives. Enemas can prove useful in cases of impaction or unresponsive constipation

Summary

- Untreated or unrecognised CIGH can lead to rare but rapidly fatal consequences, including bowel perforation or necrosis, aspiration from faecal vomiting or infection from faecal stasis.
- Monitoring for gastrointestinal adverse effects is as important as other physical health parameters.
- It is vital to treat assertively any emerging constipation and refer for immediate specialist advice if initial treatment does not work or symptoms are worsening.
- Non-drug treatments are useful in reducing the risk of constipation and include increasing exercise, ensuring adequate fluid intake, increasing dietary fibre.
- Avoid concurrent medication which can exacerbate the risk of constipation (e.g. opioids, anti-diarrhoeal and anticholinergic medication).
- In uncomplicated cases of constipation, a simple bulk forming laxative or mild osmotic laxative may prove useful.
- In cases of sudden onset or deteriorating physical health, immediate use of potent stimulant and osmotic laxatives, often as enemas, is warranted.

Further reading and resources

Palmer S, McLean R, Ellis P, Harrison-Woolrych M (2005) Life Threatening Clozapine induced Gastrointestinal hypomotility: An analysis of 102 cases. *J Clin Psychiatry* 2005; **69:** 5

World Gastroenterology Organisation Practice Guidelines: on Constipation.

Available at: http://www.worldgastroenterology.org/
NHS Clinical knowledge summaries. Constipation in adults, January 2008. Available at: http://www.cks.nhs.uk

References

1. Palmer S, McLean R, Ellis P, Harrison-Woolrych M. Life threatening clozapine induced gastrointestinal hypomotility: An analysis of 102 cases. *J Clin Psychiatry* 2005; **69:** 5
2. Hayes G, Gibler B. Clozapine-induced constipation. *Am J Psychiatry* 1995; **152:** 298
3. Drew L, Herdson P. Clozapine and constipation: a serious issue. *Aust N Z J Psychiatry* 1997; **31:** 149–50
4. Eronen M, Putkonen H, Hallikainen T, Vartianinen H. Lethal gastroenteritis associated with clozapine and loperamide. *Am J Psychiatry* 2003; **160:** 2242–43
5. Shammi C, Remingtin G. Clozapine-induced necrotizing colitis. *J Clin Psychopharmacol* 1997; **17:** 230–1
6. Levin T, Barrett J, Mendelowitz A. Death from clozapine-induced constipation. Case report and literature review. *Psychosomatics* 2002; **43:** 71–2
7. Hibbard K, Propst A, Frank D, Wyse J. Fatalities associated with clozapine-related constipation and bowel obstruction: A literature review and two case reports. *Psychosomatics* 2009; **50:** 416–19
8. Townsend G, Curtis D. Case report: rapidly fatal bowel ischaemia on clozapine treatment. *BMC Psychiatry* 2006; **6:** 43
9. Medicines and Healthcare products regulatory Authority. Drug Analysis Prints (DAP) Clozapine . Available at: http://www.mhra.gov.uk (accessed 2 June 2013)
10. Committee on Safety of Medicine, Medicines Control Agency. Clozapine (Clozaril) and gastrointestinal obstruction. *Curr Probl Pharmacovigilance* 1999; **25:** 5
11. World Health Organization. Clozapine can impair motility of the entire GI tract. *WHO Drug Information* 2007; **21:** 93
12. World Health Organization. Clozapine and life-threatening gastrointestinal hypomotility. *WHO Drug Information* 2011; **25:** 29–30
13. Dworkin RH. Pain insensitivity in schizophrenia: a neglected phenomenon and some implications. *Schizophr Bull* 1994; **20:** 235–48
14. National Health Service. *Live well. Healthy living for everyone.* Available at: http://www.nhs.uk (accessed 20 September 2011)
15. Flanagan R, Ball R. Gastrointestinal hypomotility: An under-recognised life-threatening adverse effect of clozapine. *Forensic Sci Int* 2011; **206:** e31–36
16. Seller C, Koen L, Niehas D. Clozapine-induced intestinal obstruction — a critical examination of four cases. *South Afr J Psychiatry* 2006; **12:** 21–4
17. BNF 62. *British National Formulary.* 62nd edn. London: British Medical Association and Royal Pharmaceutical Society, 2011
18. NHS Clinical knowledge summaries. Constipation in adults, January 2008. Available at: www.cks.nhs.uk (accessed 20 September 2011)
19. Fayad S, Bruijnzeel D. A fatal case of adynamic ileus following initiation of clozapine. *Am J Psychiatry* 2012; **169:** 538–9

5.6: Urinary incontinence

Urinary incontinence is a widespread problem in people with schizophrenia and was described long before the use of antipsychotics[1]. Several first and second generation antipsychotics have been reported to worsen or cause urinary incontinence[2, 3]. Clozapine has been strongly linked to incontinence in a number of case reports and larger studies[4, 5]. Although most commonly reported to occur at night, enuresis may also occur during the day and be either stress or urge-type incontinence[6]. The incidence is not established but most studies suggest 20[3]–30%[7] (ranges from less than 1[8]–42%[9]) of clozapine users are affected. Although early spontaneous remission of symptoms has been reported[10], most of the literature suggests urinary incontinence persists in the long term [5, 6].

How clozapine causes urinary incontinence is unclear, however, maintaining continence involves multiple physiological systems, many of which are affected by clozapine. The anticholinergic properties of clozapine could inhibit detrusor contraction, leading to retention of urine and overflow[3]. Central dopamine and peripheral alpha-adrenergic blockade may cause uretheral relaxation leading to incontinence[2]. Other adverse reactions of clozapine which may contribute include sedation, lowering of seizure threshold, diabetes mellitus (causing polyuria) and diabetes insipidus[3]. Of note is that the specific α_{1a}-adrenoceptor gene polymorphism has not been shown to have a major role in clozapine-induced urinary incontinence[11].

Specific risk factors for developing clozapine-induced urinary incontinence are unclear, however *Table 5.6.1* shows risk factors for the general population, which may help identify those who need closer monitoring.

Identification

The first challenge is to identify accurately those who develop clozapine-induced urinary incontinence. Many will be reluctant to report this immensely embarrassing condition which can, in addition, contribute to social isolation and non-concordance. Direct questioning on bladder function should be a routine part of clozapine physical health monitoring, both before treatment and regularly thereafter. Engaging family and carers to report concerns is important and healthcare staff should be alert for soaked clothes, wet bedding or a urine smell. Other possible causes of urinary

Table 5.6.1: General risk factors for developing urinary incontinence from any cause[12, 13]

- Female
- Old age
- Increased body mass index
- Past obstetric events
- Frequent urinary infections
- History of stroke or prostatectomy

incontinence should be ruled out (e.g. urinary infection, water intoxication, poor mobility or motivation), and actively treated where appropriate. A urinalysis may also help identify confounding factors. Although it is unclear if clozapine-induced urinary incontinence is dose-related, reducing or altering the timing of clozapine may be useful to avoid periods of deep sedation.

Treatment

A variety of drug approaches have been used to resolve clozapine-induced urinary incontinence (*Table 5.6.2*). Most are reported as case reports or case series and none is without potential, further complications. Desmopressin nasal spray, one or two puffs at night is probably the most used treatment in practice, but requires close monitoring of plasma sodium levels and fluid intake to avoid hyponatremia. *Figure 5.6.1* suggests a pragmatic approach to treating clozapine-induced urinary incontinence.

Non-drug approaches include voiding last thing before retiring to bed, avoiding fluids in the evening, using an alarm during the night to aid detection of inadvertent micturition and using incontinence pads.

Figure 5.6.1: A pragmatic approach to treating clozapine-induced urinary incontinence

Before treatment:

Investigate baseline bladder function and address any underlying contributing comorbidities. Educate the patient, family or carer to report symptoms. During treatment: monitor for urinary incontinence monthly for the first 3 months, then regularly depending on clinical need. Be alert for a urine smell, soaked clothes or wet bedding

Clozapine-induced urinary incontinence confirmed

- Assess severity, frequency, time of day, impact on quality of life
- Investigate and treat comorbidities such as urinary infections, water intoxication, poor mobility or motivation
- Consider if the dose of clozapine can be decreased or manipulated (dependent on response, risk of relapse and plasma levels if appropriate)

Use non-drug approaches, if appropriate

- Voiding before retiring to bed
- Avoiding fluids in the evening
- Using an alarm during the night to aid detection of micturition
- Incontinence pads

If symptoms distressing and persistent

- Start desmopressin nasal spray, one puff (10mcgs) at night, increase to two puffs (one in each nostril) if necessary after one week
- Monitor baseline sodium levels, fluid intake, BP and weight. Repeat weekly for the first month, then every 3 months

Table 5.6.2: Pharmacological treatments used in clozapine-induced urinary incontinence

Drug (oral unless otherwise specified)	Dose	Evidence based/comment
Amitriptyline	25mg at night	Praharaj et al, 2006[14], case report, n=1, rapid resolution of enuresis was seen after four days May worsen constipation and sedation (*Chapter* 5.5)
Aripiprazole	10mg/day	Lee et al, 2010[15], case report, n=2, reported to take many months to work, multiple confounding factors reported with the cases. Enuresis returned following aripiprazole discontinuation
Desmopressin 10mcgs nasal spray	One or two puffs at night	Aronowitz et al, 1995[8], case report, n=1, rapid, complete resolution of symptoms reported Steingard, 1994[16] case report, n=1, the nocturnal enuresis completely resolved with desmopressin Frankenbury et al, 1996[4], case series, n=4, responded well, no adverse effects were seen Lurie et al, 1997[17], case reports, n=2, complete resolution of symptoms Shriqui C, 1993[18], case report, n=1, remained effective for 18 months A case of severe hyponatremia, requiring ICU admission, has been reported 1 day after starting desmopressin nasal spray[19] Close monitoring of sodium levels and fluid intake required. Increasing blood pressure and weight may indicate fluid overload
Ephedrine	25–150mg either once at night or in divided doses	Fuller et al, 1996[7], case series, n=17, 13 had a complete response of enuresis, three had a partial response, one failed to respond to ephedrine. Response continued over 12 months Ephedrine misuse is widely reported due to its CNS stimulating action. Other common adverse reactions include tachycardia, anxiety, restlessness and insomnia
Oxybutynin	5–15 mg /day	Frankenbury et al, 1996[4], case series, n=5, responded well, reported to be well tolerated Lurie et al, 1997[17], case reports, n=5, complete resolution of symptoms May worsen constipation (*Chapter* 5.5)
Trihexylphenidyl	5mg at night	Pojurovsky et al, 1996[20], case report, n=2, response continued for the 5 weeks of follow-up
Verapamil	40–80mg/day	Pojurovsky et al, 1995[21], case report, n=1, complete resolution of symptoms reported and continued for 2 months follow-up Intensive ECG, pulse and blood pressure monitoring required

Summary

- Clozapine-induced urinary incontinence is common, under-reported and may be persistent.
- Non-drug approaches include voiding before retiring to bed, avoiding fluids in the evening, using an alarm during the night to aid micturition and incontinence pads.
- The evidence base supporting which medication to use for clozapine-induced urinary incontinence is often based on case reports or case series.
- Desmopressin nasal spray is occasionally used but sodium levels and fluid intake must be closely monitored.

References

1. Bonney W, Gupta S, Hunter R, Arndt S. Bladder dysfunction in schizophrenia. *Schizophr Res* 1997; **25:** 243–9
2. Tsakiris P, Oelke M, Michel M. Drug-induced urinary incontinence. *Drugs Aging* 2008; **25:** 541–49
3. Harrison-woolrych M, Skegg K, Ashton J, Herbiso P, Skegg D. Nocturnal enuresis in patients taking clozapine, risperidone, olanzapine and quetiapine: comparative cohort study. *Br J Psychiatry* 2011;**199:** 140–4
4. Frankenburg F, Kando J, Centorrino F, Gilbert J. Bladder dysfunction associated with clozapine therapy. *J Clin Psychiatry* 1996; **57:** 39–40
5. Lin C, Bai Y, Chen C Lan T. A retrospective study of clozapine and urinary incontinence in Chinese in-patients. *Acta Psychiatr Scand* 1999; **100:** 158–61
6. Jeong S, Kim J, Ahn Y, Lee K, Kim SW, Jung D, Kim Y. A 2-year prospective follow up study of lower urinary tract symptoms in patients treated with clozapine. *J Clin Psychopharmacol* 2008; **28:** 618–24
7. Fuller M, Borovicka M, Jaskiw G, Simon M, Kwon K, Koniciki E. Clozapine-induced urinary incontinence: Incidence and treatment with ephedrine. *J Clin Psychiatry* 1996; **57:** 514–8
8. Aronowitz J, Safferman A. Lieberman J. Management of clozapine-induced enuresis. *Am J Psychiatry* 1995; **152:** 472
9. Agarwal V. Urinary incontinence with risperidone. *J Clin Psychiatry* 2000; **61:** 219
10. Warner J, Harvey C, Barnes T. Clozapine and urinary incontinence. *Int Clin Psychopharmacol* 1994; **9:** 207–9
11. Hsu JW, Wang YC, Lin CC, Bai YM, Chen JY, Chiu HJ, et al. No evidence for association of Alpha 1α adrenoceptor gene polymorphism and clozapine-induced urinary incontinence. *Neuropsychobiology* 2000; **42:** 62–5
12. Bortolitti A, Bernardini B, Colli E, Benedetto P. Nacci G, Landoni M, et al. Prevalence and risk factors for urinary incontinence in Italy. *Eur Urol* 2000; **37:** 128–9
13. Ueda T, Tmaki M, Kageyama A, Yoshimura N, Yoshida O. Urinary incontinence among community-dwelling people aged 40 years or older in Japan: Prevalence, risk factors, knowledge and self-perception. *Int J Urol* 2000; **7:** 95–103
14. Praharaj SK, Arora M. Amitriptyline for clozapine-induced nocturnal enuresis and sialorrhea. *Br J Clin Pharmacol* 2005; **63:** 128–9

15. Lee MJ, Kim CE. Use of aripiprazole in clozapine induced enuresis: Report of two cases. *J Korean Med Sci* 2010; **25:** 333–5
16. Steingard S. Use of desmopressin to treat clozapine-induced nocturnal enuresis. *J Clin Psychiatry* 1994; **55:** 315–6
17. Lurie S, Hosmer C. Oxybutynin and intranasal desmopressin for clozapine-induced urinary incontinence. *J Clin Psychiatry* 1997; **58:** 404
18. Shriqui C. Treatment of clozapine-induced enuresis with desmopressin. *Schizophr Res* 1993; **9:** 251
19. Sarma S, Ward W, O'Brien J, Frost A, Iwaniak J. Severe hyponatraemia associated with desmopressin nasal spray to treat clozapine-induced nocturnal enuresis. *Aust N Z J Psychiatry* 2005; **39:** 949
20. Pojurovski M, Modai I, Mark M, Weizman A. Trihexyphenidyl as a possible therapeutic option in clozapine-induced nocturnal enuresis. *Int Clin Psychopharmacol* 1996; **11:** 61–3
21. Pojurovski M, Schneidman M, Mark M, Weizman A. Verapamil treatment in clozapine-induced sleep-related enuresis: a case report. *Eur Psychiatry* 1995; **10:** 413–15

5.7: Hypersalivation

Clozapine-induced hypersalivation (CIH), also called sialorrhea or ptyalism, occurs frequently at a rate of approximately 30%[1] (the reported incidence ranges from 30–80%)[2]. It usually develops early on in treatment, can be persistent, worse at night and can be the cause of much social isolation and increased prejudice. Further consequences of CIH include sleep disturbances, swelling of the salivary glands, parotitis, skin irritation or infection and early discontinuation of treatment[1,3]. Most worrying is the possible but rare association with aspiration pneumonia which can be life-threatening[4,5]. Prompt treatment is essential to prevent the medical and psychosocial consequences of CIH.

Pathophysiology of CIH

The exact mechanism underlying CIH is unknown, although a variety of theories are proposed. Salivary flow is mainly under cholinergic parasympathetic control through muscarinic M_3 and M_4 receptors. The adrenergic sympathetic system also has a minor effect increasing protein levels in saliva[1,3]. Cholinergic M_3 and M_4 receptors exert opposing effects, with M_3 blockade and M_4 stimulation increasing salivation. Clozapine is an antagonist at M_3 receptors and a full or partial agonist at M_4 receptors, and thus may mimic endogenous controls to increase salivation. This is in part supported by the observation that pirenzepine, a selective M_1 and M_4 muscarinic antagonist, may be a treatment option for CIH. Adrenergic $alpha_1$ and $alpha_2$ receptors are also present on the salivary glands, and some (but not all) $alpha_2$ antagonists such as clozapine cause hypersalivation[1]. Centrally acting $alpha_2$ receptor agonists such as clonidine, lofexidine and guanfacine have some limited support in treating CIH. There is doubt, however, that clozapine increases salivation at all and the fault lies with an altered swallowing reflex or a disturbance in the normal circadian pattern of salivary flow. Data from saliva flow rate studies which compared patients taking clozapine against controls have failed to show any difference in flow rate, volume or composition[6,7]. However, in both studies, saliva samples were taken during the day and involved few patients (26 patients in total).

It is likely that multiple factors are involved in CIH, which probably varies in individuals. This may account for the persistent and difficult to treat symptoms experienced by some.

Assessment of CIH

In clinical practice it is often difficult to assess the extent of CIH or the effectiveness of treatment. The most accurate methods such as cannulation of the salivary glands or collecting whole saliva are impractical. However, a simple rating scale such as the

5-point Nocturnal Hypersalivation Rating Scale (NHRS) or the Drooling Severity Scale (DSS) can be useful (*Table 5.7.1*)[1,8]. Estimating the diameter of wetness on a pillow or tissue paper placed over the pillow may also give a rough guide as to the severity of nocturnal hypersalivation[1].

Table 5.7.1: Subjective rating scales for monitoring CIH

The 5-point Nocturnal Hypersalivation Rating Scale (NHRS)
Rate symptom severity based on patient and clinician observations 0= Absent, no hypersalivation 1= Minimal (signs of saliva on the pillow in the morning) 2= Mild (hypersalivation wakes the patient up once during the night) 3= Moderate (hypersalivation wakes the patient up twice during the night) 4= Severe (hypersalivation wakes the patient up at least 3 times during the night)
The Drooling Severity Scale (DSS)
Rate symptom severity based on patient and clinician observations 1= Never drools, dry 2= Mild, only wet lips 3= Moderate, wet on lips and chin 4= Severe clothing becomes wet 5= Profuse, clothing, hands and objects become wet

Non-drug treatments

Any patient reporting CIH should be treated promptly with pharmacological intervention. However, the following non-drug treatments may also be considered. Chewing of sugar-free gum during the day can be useful as it encourages patients to swallow and is socially acceptable. Sleeping at night on several pillows can help in those who are regularly woken by a chocking sensation and placing a towel on the pillow can also help prevent soaking of clothes[1]. Educating the patient before starting clozapine and reinforcing during treatment is important and can alleviate some of the fear associated with this distressing adverse reaction.

Pharmacological treatments

There is no medication currently licensed for CIH. The current evidence base supporting which treatments to use in CIH is often derived from case reports or case series[2]. In an attempt to guide practice, *Figure 5.7.1* provides a pragmatic treatment approach based on the most widely used strategies in the UK. The drugs which have been used for CIH can be classed as either selective or non-selective anticholinergic agents, $alpha_2$ receptor agonists, substituted benzamide derivatives or miscellaneous agents. *Table 5.7.2* provides the current limited evidence base supporting the treatment choices. Hyoscine hydrobromide tablets, despite having no supporting evidence, are widely used and should probably be the first treatment choice. It is important to advise patients to chew or suck the tablets to induce a local action, and to remember to look out for anticholinergic adverse effects such as constipation, urinary retention, blurred vision, drowsiness and dizziness, all of which can be exacerbated with clozapine. If hyoscine is ineffective or only partial effective, pirenzepine may be a suitable alternative. Pirenzepine is either unlicensed or no longer marketed in many countries including the UK and United States, but it is

Figure 5.7.1: A pragmatic approach for treating CIH

Before treatment: Educate the patient, family and carers on the symptoms and risks associated with CIH
During treatment: Monitor for CIH at least weekly for the first month, then monthly for the first 3 months. Subsequent monitoring should be dependent on the individual and discussions with the clinical team

CIH diagnosed

- Assess severity, frequency, time of day, impact on quality of life. Consider using the NHRS or DSS rating scales
- Investigate comorbidities, such as respiratory problems which may increase the risk of complications
- Consider if the dose of clozapine can be decreased (dependent on response, risks of relapse and plasma levels if appropriate)

↓

Use non-drug approaches if appropriate: chewing gum, elevating pillows, placing a towel on the pillow

↓

Hyoscine hydrobromide tablets 300mcgs at night — ensure that the patient sucks or chews the tablet. Consider increasing the dose (in weekly increments) up to a maximum of 900mcgs daily, depending on response and tolerability.
Usually given three times a day or a larger dose at night

↓

Assess response over one month, or sooner in more severe symptoms

Partial response	No response
↓	↓
Add	Discontinue and switch to

↓

Pirenzepine tablets 50mg at night, increasing to 150mg daily (in divided doses) if required

Assess response over a month, or sooner in more severe cases. If partial or no-response, consider augmenting or switching to an alternative option from *Table* 5.7.2. Monitor for side-effects which may be exacerbated with the treatment choice and clozapine

usually available through an import company on a named patient basis. Pirenzepine does not cross the blood brain barrier, so central anticholinergic adverse effects such as confusion and dizziness are uncommon, although other adverse effects are similar to hyoscine hydrobromide. If both hyoscine and pirenzepine do not provide adequate relief from CIH, a trial of an alternative treatment from *Table 5.7.2* is tentatively recommended based on clinician and patient preference.

Table 5.7.2: Pharmacological treatments used in CIH

(No drug is currently licensed in the UK for CIH)

Drug	Dose	Evidence base/comment
Anticholinergics: note clozapine has prominent anticholinergic effects which can be enhanced when combining with an anticholinergic. Monitor especially for constipation, urinary retention and cognitive impairment		
Amitriptyline tablets	25mg at night	Praharaj et al, 2007[9], case report, n=1, 25mg at night, marked reduction of CIH reported Copp et al, 1991[10], case reports, n=4, 75–100mg daily, reported resolution of symptoms in all four patients, did not report on adverse reactions of the combination Should not be routinely used. Potential increase in anticholinergic, sedative, cardiac adverse effects and increased risk of seizures if given concurrently with clozapine
Atropine eye drops 1%	1–2 drops sublingually at night	Sharma et al, 2004[11], case report, n=1, used two drops of 1% solution twice daily then swallowed, complete resolution of CIH within 2 weeks. No adverse effects reported Comley et al, 2000[12], case report, n=1, 1–2 drops in the morning resulted in resolution of hypersalivation throughout the day Antonello et al, 1999[13], case report, n=3, one drop of 1% solution given at bedtime, allow a further one drop in a glass of water if required, immediate relief in all patients, beneficial effect was short-lived Often short-acting, rebound hypersalivation may occur in the early hours of the morning, can be either dropped directly under the tongue or made into a solution with water
Benzotropine tablets	2mg daily	Bourgeois et al, 1991[14], case report, n=1, limited details but reported effective and well tolerated
Glycopyrrolate tablets	4–8mg daily	Robb et al, 2008[15], case reports, n=3, adolescent females with CIH, improvement reported in all, one adverse reaction of constipation, one report of dry mouth

Table 5.7.2: Pharmacological treatments used in CIH *continued*

Drug	Dose	Evidence base/comment
Glycopyrrolate tablets, *continued*	4–8mg daily	Duggal 2007[16], case report, n=1, reduction in CIH reported after two days, which was dose dependent, constipation worsened Glycopyrrolate does not cross the blood brain barrier so central anticholinergic effects are unlikely
Hyoscine hydrobromide tablets Patches	300–900mcgs at night or in divided doses 1.5mg every 72 hours	No published evidence currently exists, however widely used in the UK Gaftanyuk et al, 2004[17] reported a single case, CIH resistant to tolterodine, clonidine patch and benzotropine. CIH resolved within hours of starting the patch and the effect persisted for several months McKane et al, 2001[18], case reports, n=4, well tolerated, dramatic improvement, no details given
Ipratropium Bromide nasal spray 0.03%	2 sprays sublingually at night (up to 2 sprays 3 times a day of the 0.06% has been used)	Socalingam et al, 2009[19], RCT, n=20, no difference between placebo or ipratropium after 2 weeks, low ipratropium dose, subjective measures used, large placebo effect recorded Freudenreich et al, 2004[20], case series, n=9, seven had a full or partial response, although effect wore off after a few hours (between 2–8 hours) Tessier et al, 2001[21], case series, n=10, all patients subjectively reported an improvement or resolution of nocturnal symptoms over 6 months Calderon et al, 2000[22], case series, n=10, 0.03% one spray into each nostril at bedtime, eight reported a response, one discontinued treatment due to dry nostrils and mucosal bleed, six reported continuing response at 6-month follow-up Ipratropium was reported to be well tolerated in the above studies and appears to have minimal systemic absorption
Pirenzepine tablets	50–150mg at night or in divided doses	Schneider et al, 2004[23], pilot study, n=29, 50mg per day for 3 days added. Reports of CIH reduced from 69–35%, with the addition of pirenzepine, no changes in clozapine or norclozapine levels were reported because of pirenzepine Bai et al, 2001[24], RCT, n=20, pirenzepine 100mg/ day versus placebo for 8 weeks, evaluated by measuring the diameter of wetted area on tissue paper over the pillow. CIH reduced by 15.6% with pirenzepine but was not significant versus placebo

Table 5.7.2: Pharmacological treatments used in CIH *continued*

Drug	Dose	Evidence base/comment
Pirenzepine tablets, *continued*	50–150mg at night or in divided doses	Fritze et al, 1995[25], case series, n=120, pirenzepine 25–100mg daily, clinical observations reported successful treatment, only adverse effect noted was mild diarrhoea Unlicensed product in the UK, United States and Canada. It does not cross the blood brain barrier so central anticholinergic effects are unlikely. Up to 150mg per day of pirenzepine has been used in other indications
Trihexyphenidyl	5–15mg at night	Spivak et al, 1997[8], case series, n=14, 44% reduction in nocturnal CIH by day 12 Aggarwal et al, 2009[26], case report, n=1, used 6mg in divided doses, response reported
Oxybutynin immediate release	Up to 15mg daily in divided doses	Leung et al, 2011[27], single case report. Improved from DSS of 5 to 2
Alpha 1 agonists – should be used with caution because of the increased risk of postural hypotension when co-administered with clozapine		
Clonidine patch	0.1mg–0.2mg daily	Grabowski et al, 1992[28], case reports, n=4, two showed a sustained improvement, one a limited improvement, one no improvement Clonidine patch is not routinely available
Clonidine Tablets	50–100mcgs at night	Praharaj et al, 2005[29], open labelled, naturalistic case series, n=12, initially prescribed 50mcgs at night which could be increased to 100mcg at night if no improvement at 2 weeks. Used the estimated diameter of wet pillow as a subjective marker, 11 had a partial or good response at week 4. No side-effects reported
Guanfacine Alpha2A-receptor agonist	1mg daily	Webber et al, 2004[30], case report, n=1, response seen within 4 days which persisted over 1 month
Lofexidine	0.2mg twice daly	Corrigan et al, 1995[31], case report, n=1, trialed for 1 month, persistent symptoms resolved
Substituted benzamide derivatives		
Amisulpride	100–400mg daily	Praharaj et al, 2009[32], case report, n=1, 50mg daily of amisulpride, improvement sustained to at least 3 months follow-up Kreinin et al, 2006[33], RCT, n=20, evaluated using the NHRS, significant

Table 5.7.2: Pharmacological treatments used in CIH *continued*		
Drug	Dose	Evidence base/comment
Amisulpride, *continued*	100–400mg daily	improvement seen from week 2, NHRS in the amisulpride group at 3-week endpoint was 1.40 (±1.10) versus 2.60 (±1.35) in placebo (p=0.026). 95% of patients reported an increase in prolactin during treatment with amisulpride Croissant et al, 2005[34], case report, n=1, clozapine dose was lowered when amisulpride was added leading to an almost complete resolution of hypersalivation Not available in Canada or the United States Praharaj et al, 2011[35], single case report. The DSS improved from 4 to 2 over 2 weeks. Day time hypersalivation improved more than nocturnal symptoms
Moclobemide	150–300mg daily	Kreinin et al, 2009[36], pilot open study, n=14, evaluated using the NHRS, CIH completely or partial resolved in nine (64%) of subjects at 2 weeks. Beneficial effects began after 4 days of treatment
Sulpride	150–300mg daily	Kreinin et al, 2005[37], uncontrolled trial, n=18, evaluated using the NHRS, at the end of 3 weeks 15 achieved a full response and three continued to experience mild hypersalivation Not available in Canada or the United States
Others		
Botulinum toxin-A injection (BTX)	Bilateral parotid gland injections (150 IU into each gland)	Kahl et al, 2004[38], case report, n=1, reduction in CIH seen within 2 weeks and lasted for more than 12 weeks. Several RCTs support BTX in sialorrhea secondary to Parkinson's disease. Complications such as jaw dislocation possible[3]
Bupropion tablets	100–150mg daily	Stern et al, 2009[39], case report, n=1, patient had very limited response to other medicines for CIH, day time hypersalivation improved within a few days, CIH still present at night Can lower the seizure threshold which may be a concern with clozapine
Combination trials		
Benzatropine + Terazosin in combination or individually	Benzatropine 1mg twice daily Terazosin 2mg at night	Reinstein et al, 1999[40], retrospective, open label, non-randomised, n=60, 4 treatment arms, including no treatment. Those on no treatment (n=15), four (26.7%) discontinued clozapine because of CIH and a further 33% showed either a tolerance or improvement to CIH at week 12. The percentage of patients who showed complete remission of CIH at the 12-week endpoint were 10 (66.7%) in the benzatropine-only group, 14 (93.3%) in the terazosin-only group, and 15 (100%) in the combination group

Table 5.7.2: Pharmacological treatments used in CIH *continued*

Drug	Dose	Evidence base/comment
Benzatropine + Terazosin in combination or individually, *continued*	Benzatropine 1mg twice daily Terazosin 2mg at night	Although terazosin appeared to be effective, it is important to remember that terazosin, similar to clozapine, is an $alpha_1$ antagonist so additive hypotensive effects may be seen with the combination
Comparative trials		
Glucopyrrolate versus biperiden	Glucopyr-rolate 1mg twice or Benperiden 2mg twice daily	Liang et al, 2010[41], small, randomised, double blind cross-over study, n=12, 4 weeks on each preparation, evaluated using the DRS. Glycopyrrolate produced the greatest reduction in DRS with no change in cognition, response seen within 1 week of treatment
Amisulpride vs moclobemide	Amisulpride 400mg/day Moclobemide 300mg/day	Kreinin et al, 2011[42]. 6-week, open-labeled, fixed dose study (n=53). Both amisulpride and moclobemide proved effective. 74% responded to amisulpride, 83% responded to moclobemide

Summary

- Clozapine induced hypersalivation (CIH) is one of the most common and troublesome side-effects associated with clozapine.
- Prompt treatment is essential to prevent the medical and psychosocial consequences of CIH.
- Non-drug treatment such as chewing sugar-free gum, elevating bed pillows and covering the pillow with a towel can be useful in conjunction with pharmaceutical approaches.
- A simple hypersalivation rating scale can help assess severity and response to treatment.
- The evidence base supporting which medication to use for CIH is often based on case reports or case series.
- Hyoscine hydrobromide and pirenzepine are commonly used, but similar to other anticholinergics can exacerbate side-effects such as constipation, urinary retention, and blurred vision when given concurrently with clozapine.

References

1. Praharaj SK, Arora M, Gandorra S (2006) Clozapine-induced sialorrhea: Pathophysiology and management strategies. *Psychopharmacology* **185:** 265–73

2. Syed R, Au K, Cahill C, et al. Pharmacological interventions for clozapine induced hypersalivation.

Cochrane Database of Systematic Reviews 2008, Issue 3, Art, No.: CD005579. DOI: 10.1002/14651858.CD005579.pub2

3. Sockalingam S, Shammi C, Remington G. Clozapine-induced hypersalivation: A review of treatment strategies. *Can J Psychiatry* 2007; **52:** 377–84
4. Hinkes R, Quesada TV, Currier MB, et al (1996) Aspiration pneumonia possibly secondary to clozapine-induced sialorrhea. *J Clin Psychopharmacol* **16:** 462–3
5. Taylor D, Douglas-Hall P, Olofinjana B, et al (2009) Reasons for discontinuing clozapine: matched, case-control comparison with risperidone long-acting injection. *Br J Psychiatry* **194:** 165–7
6. Rabinowitz T, Frankenburg FR, Centorrino F, et al (1996) The effect of clozapine on saliva flow rate: a pilot study. *Biol Psychiatry* **40:** 1132–34
7. Ben-Aryeh H, Jungerman T, Szargel R, et al. Salivary flow-rate and composition in schizophrenia patients on clozapine: subjective reports and laboratory data. *Biol Psychiatry* 1996; **39:** 946–9
8. Spivak B, Adlersberg S, Rosen L, et al. Trihexyphenidyl treatment of clozapine-induced hypersalivation. *Int Clin Psychopharmacol* 1997; **12:** 213–5
9. Praharaj S.K, Arora M. Amitriptyline for clozapine-induced nocturnal enuresis and sialorrhea. *Br J Clin Pharmacol* 2005; **63:** 128–9
10. Copp PJ, Lament R, Tennant TG. Amitriptyline in clozapine-induced sialorrhea. *Br J Psychiatry* 1991; **159:** 166
11. Sharma A, Ramaswamy S, Dahl E et al (2004) Intraoral application of atropine sulphate ophthalmic solution for clozapine-induced sialorrhea. Annals of Pharmacotherapy 2004; 38: 1538
12. Comley C, Galletly C, Ash D. Use of atropine eye drops for clozapine induced hypersalivation. *Aust N Z J Psychiatry* **34:** 1033–34
13. Antonello C, Tessier P. Clozapine and sialorrhea: a new intervention for this bothersome and potentially dangerous side effect. *J Psychiatry Neurosci* 1999; **24:** 250
14. Bourgeois JA, Drexler KG, Hall MJ. Hypersalivation and clozapine. *Hosp Community Psychiatry* 1991; **42:** 1174
15. Robb AS, Lee RH, Cooper EB, et al. Glycopyrrolate for treatment of clozapine-induced sialorrhea in three adolescents. *J Child Adolesc Psychopharmacol* 2008; **18:** 99–107
16. Duggal HS. Glycopyrrolate for clozapine-induced sialorrhea. *Prog Neuropsychopharmacol Biol Psychiatry* 2007; **31:** 1546–47
17. Gaftanyuk O, Trestman RL. Scopolamine patch for clozapine-induced sialorrhea. *Psychiatr Serv* 2004; **55:** 318
18. McKane JP, Hall C, Akram G. Hyoscine patches in clozapine-induced hypersalivation. *Psychiatr Bull* 2001; **25:** 277
19. Socalingam S, Shammi C, Remmington G. Treatment of clozapine-induced hypersalivation with ipratropium bromide: A randomized, double-blind, placebo-controlled crossover study. *J Clin Psychiatry* 2009; **70:** 1114–19
20. Freudenreich O, Beebe M, Goff DC. Clozapine-induced sialorrhea treated with sublingual ipratropium spray: a case series. *J Clin Psychopharmacol* 2004; **24:** 98–100
21. Tessier P, Antonello C. Clozapine and sialorrhea: Update. *J Psychiatry Neurosci* 2001; **26:** 253
22. Calderon J, Rubin E, Sobota WL. Potential use of ipatropium bromide for the treatment of clozapine-induced hypersalivation: A preliminary report. *Int Clin Psychopharmacol* 2000; **15:** 49–52
23. Schneider B, Weigmann H, Hiemke C, et al. (Reduction of clozapine-induced hypersalivation by

pirenzepine is safe. *Pharmacopsychiatry* 2004; **37:** 43–5
24. Bai YM, Lin CC, Chen JY, et al. Therapeutic effect of pirenzepine for clozapine-induced hypersalivation: a randomized, double-blind, placebo-controlled, cross-over study. *J Clin Psychopharmacol* 2001; **21:** 608–11
25. Fritze J, Elliger T. Pirenzepine for clozapine-induced hypersalivation. *Lancet* 1995; **346:** 1034
26. Aggarwal A, Garg A, Jiloha R. Trihexphenidyl (benzhexol) in clozapine-induced nocturnal enuresis and sialorrhea. *Indian J Med Sci* 2009; **63:** 470–1
27. Leung J, Puri N, Jacobson M. Immediate release oxybutynin for the treatment of clozapine-induced sialorrhea. *Ann Pharmacother* 2011; **45:** e45
28. Grabowski J. Clonidine treatment of clozapine-induced hypersalivation. *J Clin Psychopharmacol* 1992; **12:** 69–70
29. Praharaj S.K, Verm P, Roy D, et al. Is clonidine useful for treatment of clozapine-induced sialorrhea? *J Psychopharmacol* 2005; **19:** 426–8
30. Webber MA, Szwast SJ, Steadman TM, et al. Guanfacine treatment of clozapine-induced sialorrhea. *J Clin Psychopharmacol* 2004; **24:** 675–6
31. Corrigan FM, MacDonald S, Reynolds GP. Clozapine-induced hypersalivation and the $alpha_2$ adrenoceptor. *Br J Psychiatry* 1995; **167:** 412
32. Praharaj SK, Sarkar S, Sinha VK. Amisulpride treatment for clozapine-induced sialorrhea. *J Clin Psychopharmacol* 2009; **29:** 189–90
33. Kreinin A, Novitski D, Weizman A. Amisulpride treatment of clozapine-induced hypersalivation in schizophrenia patients: A randomized, double-blind, placebo-controlled cross-over study. *Int Clin Psychopharmacol* 2006; **21:** 99–103
34. Croissant B, Hermann D, Olbrich R. Reduction of side-effects by combining clozapine with amisulpride: Case report and short review of clozapine induced-hypersalivation. *Pharmacopsychiatry* 2005; **38:** 38–9
35. Praharj S, Ray P, Gondotra S. Amisulpride improved debilitating clozapine-induced sialorrhea. *Am J Ther* 2011; **18:** e84–e85
36. Kreinin A, Miodownik C, Libov I. Moclobemide treatment of clozapine-induced hypersalivation: Pilot open study. *Clin Neuropharmacol* 2009; **32:** 151–3
37. Kreinin A, Epshtein S, Sheinkman A, et al. Sulpiride addition for the treatment of clozapine-induced hypersalivation: Preliminary study. *Isr J Psychiatry Relat Sci* 2005; **42:** 61–3
38. Kahl KG, Hagenah J, Zapf S, et al. Botulinum toxin as an effective treatment of clozapine-induced hypersalivation. *Psychopharmacology* 2004; **173:** 229–30
39. Stern RG, Bellucci D, Cursi-Vogel N, et al. Clozapine-induced sialorrhea alleviated by bupropion-a case report. *Prog Neuropsychopharmacol Biol Psychiatry* 2009; **33:** 1578–80
40. Reinstein MJ, Sirotovskaya LA, Chasanov MA, et al. Comparative efficacy and tolerability of benzatropine and terazosin in the treatment of hypersalivation secondary to clozapine. *Clin Drug Invest* 1999; **17:** 97–102
41. Liang CS, Ho PS, Shen LJ, et al. Comparison of the efficacy and impact on cognition of glycopyrrolate and biperiden for clozapine-induced sialorrhea in schizophrenia patients: a randomized, double-blind, crossover study. *Schizophr Res* 2010; **119:** 138–44
42. Kreinin A, Miodownik C, Sokolik S, Shestakova D, Libov I, Bergman J, et al. Amisulpride versus moclobemide in treatment of clozapine-induced hypersalivation. *World J Biol Psychiatry* 2011; **12:** 620–6

5.8: Fever

Since the introduction of clozapine into clinical practice, fever has been commonly reported during the initial stages of treatment. The incidence of fever varies from 0.5–55%, a range which is largely dependent on the definition of fever used[1]. Retrospective chart reviews provide the best insight into clozapine-induced fevers (*Table 5.8.1*). Fever usually occurs within three weeks of starting clozapine and continues for between one and five days[2–5]. In the vast majority of cases, the fever spontaneously resolves, either upon a temporary suspension of clozapine or by cautiously continuing treatment. In all cases of clozapine-induced fever, it would be prudent to rule out a more sinister cause such as an underlying infection, neuroleptic malignant syndrome (NMS), agranulocytosis or myocarditis. However, there is no evidence suggesting that this early appearing fever is indicative of a dangerous comorbidity.

Table 5.8.1: Retrospective chart reviews investigating clozapine-induced fever

Author (year)	Number of patients (N)	Definition of fever	Incidence of fever, %	Onset after clozapine initiation, days	Duration of fever, days	Comment
Chung et al, 2008[2]	227	≥38°C	13.7%	13.7 (±7.1)	4.7 (±3)	77.4% were given paracetamol and showed symptomatic relief. Clozapine was stopped in 14/31 and the fever subsided spontaneously within 48 hours in most of these. Seven were successfully re-challenged with clozapine
Tham et al, 2002[3]	93	≥38.5°C	20.4%	13.8 (3–26)	3.8 (±2.6)	Medical complications were not considered to be the cause of fever in any case. 16/19 with fever had a temporary suspension of clozapine. All were successfully re-challenged without the reoccurrence of fever
Jeong et al, 2001[4]	98	≥37.5°C	43.8%	11 (5–20)	1 (±3.1)	The outcome was not reported
Nittenson et al, 1995[5]	51	>100oF (>37.7°C)	25.5%	12	2.6	Clozapine was stopped briefly in all those with a fever, then successfully re-introduced

Fever does not appear to be related to the dose of clozapine but age, the rate of titration, the presence of a physical illness and concurrent use of valproate may be implicated[2]. Of interest is that the presence of an early fever with clozapine does not affect discontinuation rates at one year[3].

Mechanism

The mechanism behind clozapine-induced fever is unclear. Theories such as an allergic reaction or mild NMS are unlikely, given that the fever does not appear to return on re-challenge and, when measured, creatine kinase (CK) levels are either normal or only mildly elevated[3,6]. Other theories suggest an immunomodulating effect of clozapine. Cytokines (which are involved in the inflammatory response) such as interleukin-6, soluble interleukin-2 receptors and tumour necrosis factor-α have been shown to be increased after two weeks of clozapine in those with a fever[7]. C-reactive protein levels[6] and granulocyte counts[7] have also been shown to be elevated in those with clozapine-induced fever, although the significance of this is unknown.

Treatment of clozapine-induced fever

Although fever associated with clozapine is usually benign and transient, other possible causes should be ruled out. Physical investigations may include a creatine kinase (CK) level, chest X-ray, urine culture and repeating routine blood tests[2]. Any concurrent cardiac symptoms (e.g. tachycardia, dyspnoea or chest pain) must provoke an immediate cessation of clozapine and an urgent referral to medical services. Assuming no concurrent comorbidity is discovered, clozapine can usually be continued with close monitoring, and the fever generally spontaneously resolves. Paracetamol (acetaminophen) appears useful to reduce temperature and ease symptoms[2]. For those with a high grade fever (e.g. >39°C), clozapine should be temporarily suspended until resolution of symptoms. Re-challenging with clozapine is usually appropriate and without incident.

Summary

- Clozapine-induced fever is common in the first three weeks of treatment. It is usually benign and often resolves in a few days.
- In all cases it would be prudent to rule out a more sinister comorbidity such as an infection, neuroleptic malignant syndrome, agranulocytosis or myocarditis.
- For those with a fever, consider either suspending clozapine (especially if >39°C) or continuing treatment cautiously.
- Paracetamol (acetaminophen) usually helps symptoms.
- Re-challenge with clozapine is usually appropriate and without incident.

References

1. Lowe C, Grube R, Scates A. Characterization and clinical management of clozapine-induced fever. *Ann Pharmacother* 2007; **41**: 1700–04

2. Chung J, Chong C, Chung K, Dunn E, Tang O, Chan W. The incidence and characteristics of clozapine-induced fever in a local psychiatric unit in Hong Kong. *Can J Psychiatry* 2008; **53**: 857–62

3. Tham J, Dickson R. Clozapine-induced fevers and 1-year clozapine discontinuation rate. *J Clin Psychiatry* 2002; **63**: 880–4

4. Jeong S, Ahn Y, Koo Y. The characteristics of clozapine-induced fever. *Schizophr Res* 2002; **56**: 191–3

5. Niteson N, Kando J, Frankenburg F, Zanarini M. Fever associated with clozapine administration. *Am J Psychiatry* 1995; **152**: 1102

6. Kohen I, Afzal N, Hussain S, Manu P. Increases in C-reactive protein may predict recurrence of clozapine-induced fever. *Ann Pharmacother* 2009; **43**: 143–6

7. Pollmacher T, Hinze-Selch D, Mullington J. Effects of clozapine on plasma cytokine and soluble cytokine receptor levels. *J Psychopharmacol* 1996; **16**: 403–9

5.9: Venous thromboembolism

Venous thromboembolism (VTE) is a rare but potentially fatal adverse reaction of antipsychotics. Second generation antipsychotics and low potency first generation antipsychotics carry a greater risk than other antipsychotics[1,2]. Clozapine appears to have the most reports[3,4] and data from the Swedish authorities suggest that the risk of VTE with clozapine is one case per 2000–6000 exposures[5]. The German and Swiss pharmacovigilance database similarly reported the VTE risk with clozapine as one in 2600 treated patients. The US Food and Drug Administration (FDA) lists the risk of a fatal pulmonary embolus with clozapine as one case per 3450 person-years of use, which is 27.5 times higher than in the general population[7].

Deep vein thrombosis (DVT) and pulmonary embolism (PE) are the most frequent type of thromboembolism reported with clozapine[4], but there is also one case report linking clozapine with cerebral venous sinus thrombosis[8]. The risk of VTE with clozapine appears to be highest in the first three months of therapy[4,5] and may not be dependant on dose[5,9], although this is disputed[4]. Further specific risk factors for developing VTE with clozapine are unclear. However, *Table 5.9.1* presents risk factors for VTE in the general population, indicating those clozapine patients who need closer monitoring.

Mechanism of action

The mechanism by which clozapine may cause thromboembolism is currently unknown. It may be linked to indirect effects such as sedation or weight gain, leading to less mobility and venous stasis, or a direct effect on coagulation or antiphospholipid antibodies[4]. Axelsson et al from Linköping University, Sweden, conducted an *in-vitro* experiment investigating platelet adhesion and aggregation of four antipsychotics (clozapine, its active metabolite N-desmethyl clozapine, olanzapine, risperidone and haloperidol). Clozapine was the only antipsychotic to significantly (although weakly) increase platelet adhesion and aggregation and reduce activated partial thromboplastin time (APTT). The reduction in APTT time with clozapine was 0.4 seconds ($p<0.01$)[14]. In a case report by Davis et al in New Jersey, a patient on long-term clozapine developed antiphospolipid antibodies[15]. In this particular case, the specific class and combination of antiphospolipid antibodies may have contributed to a gross haematuria[15]. Alternative combinations of antiphospolipid antibodies however, are present in a variety of hypercoagulable disease states such as systemic lupus erythematosus. In a further, interesting Chinese study, 50 clozapine patients were matched against controls and serum antiphospholipids were measured and compared. The clozapine group showed higher levels of antiphospholipids than controls (although not significant), and the specific isotope IgM aCL was associated with higher clozapine levels. This study also discovered that un-medicated patients with schizophrenia displayed higher levels of antiphospholipids (isotope IcG aCL) than controls[16].

As the cause of venous thromboembolism is probably multifactorial, it is likely that a number of the above processes are involved.

Treatment and prevention

Treatment of VTE begins with the appropriate and timely identification of those at risk of an episode. Those at a low risk should be encouraged to have regular physical exercise and adequate fluid intake. As risk increases when one or more of the risk factors in *Table 5.9.1* is evidenced, clinicians should consider anti-embolism stockings (unless contraindicated), foot impulse devices or intermittent pneumatic compression devices (if available)[10]. Pharmacological VTE prophylaxis involves either fondaparinux, a low molecular weight heparin (caution in renal failure), or unfractionated heparin, which is continued until the risk subsides. Aspirin and other antiplatelet drugs are not adequate alone for VTE prophylaxis[10, 11]. Pharmacological treatment must be weighed against the increased risk of bleeding and thrombocytopenia associated with heparin. Many factors commonly encountered in the psychiatric patient increase bleeding risk, these include cirrhosis, hepatitis or concurrent serotonin reuptake inhibitors. There is no evidence to suggest that SSRIs reduce VTE risk in those on clozapine, but it is a theoretical possibility.

Treatment of a confirmed DVT or PE usually consists of an appropriate dose

Table 5.9.1: General population risk factors for venous thromboembolism[10, 11] (the risk of VTE significantly increases if multiple risk factors are present)

- Reduced mobility for at least 3 days* (increases the DVT risk by about tenfold)
- Medical or surgical hospitalisation
- Anaesthesia
- Surgical procedure (especially if the surgery involves the pelvis, abdomen or lower limbs)
- Central venous catheter
- Increasing age (above 60)
- Dehydration
- Known thrombophillias (e.g. prothrombin G20210A mutation[12])
- Obesity
- A significant medication comorbidity (e.g. heart or respiratory disease, cancer)
- Personal or first degree relative history of VTE
- Use of hormone replacement therapy (HRT), or the combined oral contraceptive
- Varicose veins with phlebitis
- Pregnant or puerperal

*The definition of reduced mobility in psychiatric inpatients has been suggested as the inability to walk 10 meters for 1–2 weeks[13]. Catatonia and prolonged physical restraint are notable causes of reduced mobility in psychiatry

of either fondaparinux, a low molecular weight heparin, or unfractionated heparin. This is usually followed by at least three months of a vitamin K antagonist (such as warfarin)[11, 17]. Diagnostic and treatment algorithms for venous thromboembolism have been produced by the American Institute for Clinical Systems Improvement[17] and further National treatment guidelines are available from the Scottish Intercollegiate Guidelines Network (SIGN)[11].

Clinicians should remain vigilant of the signs and symptoms of DVT and PE in clozapine patients and, if suspicious, send for immediate medical attention (*Table 5.9.2*).

Table 5.9.2: Signs and symptoms of DVT and PE[11]

Deep vein thrombosis
▸ Increased temperature ▸ Pitting oedema ▸ Prominent superficial veins ▸ Swelling ▸ Tenderness ▸ Unilateral leg pain
Pulmonary embolism
▸ Breathlessness ▸ Chest pain ▸ Collapse ▸ Focal signs in the chest ▸ Haemoptysis ▸ Hypotension ▸ Tachycardia ▸ Hypoxia cyanosis ▸ Raised jugular venous pressure ▸ Tachyponea

Post event considerations

Whether to continue or discontinue clozapine following a thromboembolic event is dependent on multiple factors and a thorough analysis of the risks and benefits of treatment. For those who have no other risk factors, have benefited greatly from clozapine and had no complications during anticoagulant treatment, continuing clozapine may be appropriate. Conversely, a life-threatening PE, coupled with poor engagement and a fluctuating mental state may warrant discontinuation of clozapine. Engaging medical colleagues, the patient, carers, pharmacy and nursing staff is essential, as is educating the patient fully about the risks and symptoms of VTE. Although alternative antipsychotics may not provide adequate stability of mental state, a high potency, first generation antipsychotic (such as haloperidol) has a lower risk of VTE[19, 20].

Summary

- Venous thromboembolism (VTE) such as a deep vein thrombosis and pulmonary embolism are rare but potentially fatal adverse reactions associated with clozapine.
- Mental health clinicians should be aware of the signs and symptoms of VTE in clozapine patients and instigate immediate medical attention if concerned.
- All clozapine patients should be advised to undertake regular physical exercise and remain fully hydrated to reduce the risk of VTE.
- Compression stockings or appropriate pharmacotherapy should be initiated in any patient with underlying risk factors of VTE.

- The decision to continue clozapine following a VTE is complex and should include the extended multidisciplinary team, patient and carer.

Further reading

Scottish Intercollegiate Guidelines Network. *Prevention and management of venous thromboembolism: A national clinical guideline*. Available at: http://www.sign.ac.uk December 2010

References

1. Parker C, Coupland C, Hippisley-Cox J. Antipsychotics drugs and risk of venous thromboembolism: nested case-control study. *Br Med J* 2010; **341:** c4245
2. Jönsson A, Horváth-Puhó, Hägg S, Pedersen L, Sørensen H. Antipsychotics and risk of venous thromboembolism: A population-based case-controlled study. *Clin Epidemiol* 2009; **1:** 19–26
3. Allenet B, Schmidlin S, Genty C, Bosson J. Antipsychotic drugs and risk of pulmonary embolism. *Pharmacoepidemiol Drug Safety* 2012; **21:** 42–8
4. Paciullo C. Evaluating the association between clozapine and venous thromboembolism. *Am J Health System Pharm* 2008; **65:** 1825–9
5. Hägg S, Spigset O, Söderström T. Association of venous thrombolism and clozapine. *Lancet* 2000; **355:** 1155–6
6. Wolstein J, Rüther E. Antipsychotic drugs and venous thromboembolism. *Lancet* 2000; **356:** 252
7. Kortepeter C, Chen M, Knudsen J, Dubitsky G, Ahmad S, Beitz J. Clozapine and venous thromboembolism. *Am J Psychiatry* 2002; **159:** 876–7
8. Werring D, Hacking D, Losseff N, Jäger H, Walsh, Foong J. Cerebral venous sinus thrombosis may be associated with clozapine. *J Neuropsychiatry Clin Neurosci* 2009; **21:** 343–5
9. Hägg S, Bate A, Stahl M, Spigset O. Association between venous thromembolism and antipsychotics. A study of the WHO database of adverse drug reactions. *Drug Safety* 2008; **31:** 685–94
10. National Institute for Health and Clinical Excellence. *Venous thromboembolism: reducing the risk. Clinical Guideline 92*. Available at: http://www.nice.org.uk . 2010.
11. Scottish Intercollegiate Guidelines Network. *Prevention and management of venous thromboembolism: A national clinical guideline*. Available at: http://www.sign.ac.uk
12. Vayá A, Lopez M, Plumé G, Ribes J. Upper-extremity deep vein thrombosis in a patient on clozapine therapy carrying the prothrombin G20210A mutation. *Pathophysiol Haemostasis Thrombosis* 2008; **36:** 105–7
13. Maly R, Masopust J, Hosak L, Konupcikova K. Assessment of risk of venous thromboembolism and its possible prevention in psychiatric patients. *Psychiatry Clin Neurosci* 2008; **62:** 3–8
14. Axelsson S, Hägg S, Eriksson A, Lindahl T, Whiss P. *In vitro* effects of antipsychotics on human platelet adhesion and aggregation and plasma coagulation. *Clin Exp Pharmacol Physiol* 2007; **34:** 775–80
15. Davis S, Kerin H, Asokan R. Antiphospholipid antibodies associated with clozapine treatment. *Am J Hematol* 1994; **46:** 166–7
16. Shen H, Li R, Xiao H, Zhou Q. Cui Q. Chen J. Higher serum clozapine level is associated with increased antiphopholipid antibodies in schizophrenia patients. *J Psychiatr Res* 2009; **43:** 615–9

17. Snow V, Qaseem A, Barry P, Hornblake R, Rodnick J, Tobolic T, et al. Management of venous thromboembolism: a clinical practice guideline from the American College of Physicians and the American Academy of Family Physicians. *Ann Internal Med* 2007; **146:** 204–210
18. Institute for Clinical Systems Improvement (ICSI). *Venous thromboembolism diagnosis and treatment.* 12 edn. January 2012. Available at: www.icsi.org
19. Srihari V, Lee T. Pulmonary embolism in a patient taking clozapine. *Br Med J* 2008; **336:** 1499–1501
20. Zhang R, Dong L, Shao F, Tan X, Ying K. Antipsychotic and venous thromboembolism risk: A meta-analysis. *Pharmacopsychiatry* 2011; **44:** 183–8

5.10: Myocarditis and cardiomyopathy

Among clozapine's numerous adverse effects, its cardiac effects are some of the most important and life-threatening. Both myocarditis and cardiomyopathy are clearly associated with clozapine treatment, although their exact incidence and timecourse are subject to some debate. What is not in doubt, however, is the potential lethality of these adverse effects. Careful, targeted monitoring is therefore essential to ensure safe use of clozapine.

Myocarditis

Causes

While there is some certainty that clozapine is a cause of myocarditis, the mechanism by which this occurs has not been determined. The timing of the onset of symptoms (see below) suggests some type of allergic reaction, possibly IgE-mediated hypersensitivity[1], although oddly, other types of allergy to clozapine (urticaria; anaphylaxis) are extremely rare. Also possible is a direct toxic effect of clozapine on cardiac tissue — a mechanism supported by the observation that the speed of titration influences the incidence of myocarditis[2] (as may genetic variations in metabolism[3]). In addition, mouse models suggest that myocarditis may arise from an excess of catecholamines in the blood, and that myocarditis may be prevented by pre-treatment with propranolol[4]. The same study also showed the potent inflammatory effects of clozapine, thereby allowing the notion that myocarditis might be brought about by both immunomodulatory and direct effects of clozapine. Certainly in humans, effects on the immune system are evidenced by fever, flu-like symptoms and changes in plasma markers of inflammation, while effects on catecholamines are also inferred from the effect of clozapine on pulse rate[3].

Post-mortem findings in subjects dying from clozapine-associated myocarditis suggest the possibility of a clozapine-induced hypereosinophilic syndrome in which eosinophils and macrophages infiltrate cardiac tissue[5].

Incidence

The reported incidence of myocarditis in clozapine-treated subjects ranges from one in 29 (3.4%) to one in 6,764 (0.015%) (*Table 5.10.1*). This huge range probably includes the true value, but where this true value lies is open to speculation. Higher incidences reported in Australia suggest either better monitoring and case identification, or a specific genetic predisposition (or both). The second of these possibilities seems unlikely given the shared heritage of the people of Australia with that of the UK, Ireland and the United States. The fatality rate also varies substantially — from fewer than one in 10 cases to 75%. These figures probably represent differences in monitoring intensity, identification and treatment.

Table 5.10.1: Estimates of the incidence of clozapine-associated myocarditis

Reference	Location	Time period	Incidence: % of patients treated	Incidence: number to treat for one case	Comments
Committee on Safety of Medicines, 1993[24]	UK	1990–1993	0.08%	1 in 1,250	Three of 4 cases fatal
Killian et al, 1999[1]	Australia	1993–1999	0.19%	1 in 500	Five of 15 cases fatal
Degner et al, 2000[25]	Germany and Switzerland	1993–1998	0.029%	1 in 3,431	Three cases in 10,263
La Grenade, 2001[21]	USA	1989–1999	0.015%	1 in 6,764	17 of 28 cases confirmed; 18 died
Hagg et al, 2001[26]	Sweden	1983–1999	0.053%	1 in 1,888	Three of 8 cases fatal
Reinders et al, 2004[27]	Australia	1993–2002	3.4%	1 in 29	Rate may have been higher. Single unit
Haas et al, 2007[28]	Australia	1993–2003	0.7–1.2%	1 in 100	116 cases, 10 fatal

Symptoms and signs

Most cases of myocarditis present with a non-specific but classic collection of symptoms, although even fatal cases of myocarditis may be otherwise symptomless. Symptoms include fever, palpitations, fatigue (each seen in patients on clozapine who do not have myocarditis), chest pain or discomfort, dyspnoea, dizziness, peripheral oedema and decreased exercise capacity[6, 7] (*Table 5.10.2*). None of these symptoms is specific to myocarditis, but some are much more common in those with the disorder: dyspnoea occurs in 90% of cases of myocarditis but is uncommon in clozapine subjects who do not have myocarditis[8]. In any patient on clozapine, symptoms of dyspnoea, palpitations and decreased exercise capacity should provoke cessation of clozapine treatment and immediate referral to specialist care.

Signs of myocarditis are also somewhat non-specific. They include hypotension, increased pulse rate, increased temperature, impaired left ventricular function, raised jugular venous pressure and ECG changes[8, 9].

Timecourse

Myocarditis can occur at any time after starting clozapine, but around 4/5 of cases are seen in the first month of treatment (*Table 5.10.3*). Median time to onset of symptoms is between 15 and 20 days. The earliest cases reported were symptomatic at three days and the latest up to 10 years after starting clozapine. Perhaps 95% or more cases will occur in the first year of treatment, with the large majority of these in the first month.

Table 5.10.2: Detecting myocarditis		
Symptoms	Signs	Investigations
Dyspnoea	Increased pulse rate	CRP>100mg/L
Palpitations	Increased respiratory rate	Troponin >2xULN
Reduced exercise tolerance	Raised jugular venous pressure	ECG – ST depression
Fever	Hypotension	Neutrophilia
Fatigue	Arrhythmia	Eosinophilia
Malaise		Echo — decreased LVF
Vomiting		
Diarrhoea		
Dizziness		
Chest pain		
Oedema		

CRP = c-reactive protein; ULN = upper limit of normal; LVF = left ventricular function

Table 5.10.3: Timecourse of myocarditis		
Reference	Timecourse: after starting clozapine	Comments
Committee on Safety of Medicines, 1993[24]	15 days to one year	Three cases only
Killian et al, 1999[1]	3–21 days	Median 15 days, 15 cases
Degner et al, 2000[25]	13–20 days	Three cases only
La Grenade, 2001[21]	14 days to 7 years	Median 21 days, 28 cases
Hagg et al, 2001[26]	3 days to 20 months	Median 16.5 days, eight cases
Reinders et al, 2004[27]	Symptoms emerged between day 11 and day 18	Mean time to onset 14.4 days, nine cases
Haas et al, 2007[28]	1 day to over a year (3285 days)	116 cases (ten — no data on timecourse) 84/106 cases occurred before day 28 (79%). Median time to onset = 17 days
Hill 2008[29]	7–3390 days	25 cases; 24 with known timecourse 80% of cases seen in first month
Ronaldson 2010[10]	14–22 days	38 cases. Mean = 17.6 days
Ronaldson 2011[30]	10–33 days	75 cases. 83% of cases occurred between days 14 and 21
Ronaldson 2012[31]	15–20 days	Five cases. Median = 19 days
Ronaldson 2012[2]	10–33 days	105 cases. Mean time to onset = 17 days

Investigations

Myocarditis cannot be definitively diagnosed without endomyocardial biopsy; a procedure not suitable for those suspected of having clozapine-induced myocarditis. Echocardiography is not invasive and can readily detect evidence of reduced cardiac function (which may or may not be a result of myocarditis). In addition to this, certain biochemical parameters are associated with myocarditis — B-type natriuretic peptide (which is rarely measured in practice), troponin I or T, C-reactive protein (CRP) may all be raised in myocarditis but all may also be normal[6, 8, 10]. Eosinophilia and neutrophilia may also be detected, but neither is specific to myocarditis nor diagnostic.

Monitoring for clozapine-induced myocarditis

Intensive monitoring of biochemical, functional and patient parameters is essential during the first month of clozapine treatment if myocarditis is to be detected and death to be avoided.

Baseline assessment ('work-up') is critical as this serves as the reference point to future measurements. Monitoring should proceed on a daily basis for patient parameters and weekly for biochemical and blood parameters. All patients will be having weekly blood samples drawn, so the additional monitoring set out in *Table 5.10.4* should present no additional burden.

Table 5.10.4: Monitoring for myocarditis

Baseline	Daily for one month	Weekly for one month
Temperature	Temperature	Full blood count
Pulse	Pulse	Troponin I or T
Blood pressure	Blood pressure	CRP
Respiratory rate	Respiratory rate	ECG
Full blood count		
Troponin I or T	Ask about:	
C-reactive protein (CRP)	Chest pain, fever, cough, shortness of breath, exercise capacity	
ECG		

Increase monitoring frequency if PR >120 or CRP or troponin slightly raised. If CRP >100mg/L or troponin >2ULN, cease clozapine. Arrhythmia and ST depression/elevation may signify myocarditis[11].

Note that this monitoring schedule will not detect all cases of myocarditis, so further vigilance is required both during the first month of treatment and afterwards.

Restarting clozapine after myocarditis

Re-exposure to clozapine after suspected myocarditis has been attempted and can be successful[9, 12, 13]. Intensive monitoring is required and clozapine titrations should be as slow as possible and begin at 6.25mg a day. Re-challenge may be unsuccessful in perhaps 50% of attempts[9], with signs and symptoms usually recurring within days of re-starting clozapine. In thirteen cases of attempted re-challenge available in the literature in 2013, no particular parameter seemed to predict success or failure, although slow re-titration was used in all but one of the successful cases. Interestingly, time to re-challenge seems not to predict success or failure[9, 14]. In one case, prescribers successfully used carvedilol and captopril to allow re-exposure to clozapine[15]. It is not clear from this single case whether or not this approach can be generally recommended.

Cardiomyopathy

By 2013 there were 58 cases of suspected clozapine-induced cardiomyopathy reported in the literature[16–20]. Estimates as to the actual incidence of cardiomyopathy in people taking clozapine have been cited as 0.02% of patients (USA figures[21]) and 0.1% of patients (Australia figures[1]) (i.e. a range of one in 1000 to one in 5000 patients). Mortality figures are not available but 11 of the 58 cases reported in the literature had a fatal outcome.

Cardiomyopathy usually presents with dyspnoea and reduced exercise capacity occurring up to seven years after starting clozapine[16–20, 22]. Echocardiography shows cardiomegaly and reduced ventricular ejection fraction. Treatment usually consists of beta-blocker and diuretics following immediate cessation of clozapine. Re-challenge has been attempted and may be successful[23]. Prophylactic ACE inhibitors may be required.

Summary

- Myocarditis and cardiomyopathy are associated with clozapine treatment.
- Myocarditis occurs mainly in the first four weeks of treatment and may present with a classic constellation of symptoms related to reduced cardiac function or may be symptomless.
- The incidence of myocarditis may be as high as one in 29 patients treated. Mortality is high.
- Monitoring of vital signs, asking about key symptoms, and testing levels of C-reactive protein and troponin are essential for the safe use of clozapine.
- Successful re-challenge after myocarditis has been reported.
- Cardiomyopathy occurs late in treatment and is much less common than myocarditis — one in 1000 patients or fewer.
- Cardiomyopathy presents with dyspnoea and reduced exercise tolerance. Mortality is lower but significant.

References

1. Killian JG, Kerr K, Lawrence C, Celermajer DS. Myocarditis and cardiomyopathy associated with clozapine. *Lancet* 1999; **354:** 1841–5
2. Ronaldson KJ, Fitzgerald PB, Taylor AJ, Topliss DJ, Wolfe R, McNeil JJ. Rapid clozapine dose titration and concomitant sodium valproate increase the risk of myocarditis with clozapine: a case-control study. *Schizophr Res* 2012; **141:** 173–8
3. Roge R, Moller BK, Andersen CR, Correll CU, Nielsen J. Immunomodulatory effects of clozapine and their clinical implications: what have we learned so far? *Schizophr Res* 2012; **140:** 204–13
4. Wang JF, Min JY, Hampton TG, Amende I, Yan X, Malek S, et al. Clozapine-induced myocarditis: role of catecholamines in a murine model. *Eur J Pharmacol* 2008; **592:** 123–7
5. Fineschi V, Neri M, Riezzo I, Turillazzi E. Sudden cardiac death due to hypersensitivity myocarditis during clozapine treatment. *Int J Legal Med* 2004; **118:** 307–9
6. Annamraju S, Sheitman B, Saik S, Stephenson A. Early recognition of clozapine-induced myocarditis. *J Clin Psychopharmacol* 2007; **27:** 479–83
7. Wooltorton E. Antipsychotic clozapine (Clozaril): myocarditis and cardiovascular toxicity. *CMAJ* 2002; **166:** 1185–6
8. Layland JJ, Liew D, Prior DL. Clozapine-induced cardiotoxicity: a clinical update. *Med J Aust* 2009; **190:** 190–2
9. Ronaldson KJ, Fitzgerald PB, Taylor AJ, McNeil JJ. Observations from 8 cases of clozapine rechallenge after development of myocarditis. *J Clin Psychiatry* 2012; **73:** 252–4
10. Ronaldson KJ, Taylor AJ, Fitzgerald PB, Topliss DJ, Elsik M, McNeil JJ. Diagnostic characteristics of clozapine-induced myocarditis identified by an analysis of 38 cases and 47 controls. *J Clin Psychiatry* 2010; **71:** 976–81
11. Magnani JW, Dec GW. Myocarditis: current trends in diagnosis and treatment. *Circulation* 2006; **113:** 876–90
12. Hassan I, Brennan A, Carroll A, Dolan M. Monitoring in clozapine rechallenge after myocarditis. *Aust Psychiatry* 2011; **19:** 370–1
13. Rosenfeld AJ, Gibbs T, Ivie R, Clarke L, Merrill DB. Successful clozapine retrial after suspected myocarditis. *Am J Psychiatry* 2010; **167:** 350–1
14. Manu P, Sarpal D, Muir O, Kane JM, Correll CU. When can patients with potentially life-threatening adverse effects be rechallenged with clozapine? A systematic review of the published literature. *Schizophr Res* 2012; **134:** 180–6
15. Rostagno C, Di NG, Placidi GF, Gensini GF. Beta-blocker and angiotensin-converting enzyme inhibitor may limit certain cardiac adverse effects of clozapine. *Gen Hosp Psychiatry* 2008; **30:** 280–3
16. Wehmeier PM, Heiser P, Remschmidt H. Myocarditis, pericarditis and cardiomyopathy in patients treated with clozapine. *J Clin Pharm Ther* 2005; **30:** 91–6
17. Roh S, Ahn DH, Nam JH, Yang BH, Lee BH, Kim YS. Cardiomyopathy associated with clozapine. *Exp Clin Psychopharmacol* 2006; **14:** 94–8
18. Makhoul B, Hochberg I, Rispler S, Azzam ZS. Dilated cardiomyopathy: an unusual complication of clozapine therapy. *Nat Clin Pract Cardiovasc Med* 2008; **5:** 566–70
19. Rostagno C, Domenichetti S, Pastorelli F, Gensini GF. Clozapine associated cardiomyopathy: a cluster

of 3 cases. *Intern Emerg Med* 2011; **6:** 281–3

20. Taneja AK, Wong J, Bayliss J. Antipsychotic-drug-induced dilated cardiomyopathy. *Br Med J Case Rep* 2009; 2009

21. La Grenade L, Graham D, Trontell A. Myocarditis and cardiomyopathy associated with clozapine use in the United States (Letter). *N Engl J Med* 2001; **345:** 224–5

22. Tanner MA, Culling W. Clozapine associated dilated cardiomyopathy. *Postgrad Med J* 2003; **79:** 412–13

23. Floreani J, Bastiampillai T. Successful re-challenge with clozapine following development of clozapine-induced cardiomyopathy. *Aust N Z J Psychiatry* 2008; **42:** 747–8

24. Committee on Safety of Medicines. Myocarditis with antipsychotics: recent cases with clozapine (Clozaril). *Curr Probl Pharmacovigilance* 1993; **19:** 9–10

25. Degner D, Bleich S, Grohmann R, Bandelow B, Ruther E. Myocarditis associated with clozapine treatment. *Aust N Z J Psychiatry* 2000; **34:** 880

26. Hagg S, Spigset O, Bate A, Soderstrom TG. Myocarditis related to clozapine treatment. *J Clin Psychopharmacol* 2001; **21:** 382–8

27. Reinders J, Parsonage W, Lange D, Potter JM, Plever S. Clozapine-related myocarditis and cardiomyopathy in an Australian metropolitan psychiatric service. *Aust N Z J Psychiatry* 2004; **38:** 915–22

28. Haas SJ, Hill R, Krum H, Liew D, Tonkin A, Demos L, et al. Clozapine-associated myocarditis: a review of 116 cases of suspected myocarditis associated with the use of clozapine in Australia during 1993–2003. *Drug Saf* 2007; **30:** 47–57

29. Hill GR, Harrison-Woolrych M. Clozapine and myocarditis: a case series from the New Zealand Intensive Medicines Monitoring Programme. *N Z Med J* 2008; **121:** 68–75

30. Ronaldson KJ, Fitzgerald PB, Taylor AJ, Topliss DJ, McNeil JJ. A new monitoring protocol for clozapine-induced myocarditis based on an analysis of 75 cases and 94 controls. *Aust N Z J Psychiatry* 2011; **45:** 458–65

31. Ronaldson KJ, Fitzgerald PB, Taylor AJ, McNeil JJ. Continuation of clozapine following mild myocarditis. *Aust N Z J Psychiatry* 2012; **46:** 910–11

5.11: Sedation and sleep architecture

Sedation is a common adverse effect of many antipsychotics. In people with agitation, restlessness or insomnia sedation can be seen as beneficial and a useful therapeutic side-effect. In others, the sedation can be prolonged or severe and reduce quality of life. Patients with sedation may show impaired cognitive or motor performance and often decide to lower or stop medication without consultation[1]. In addition, sedation increases the risk of falls and may cause weight gain by reducing activity and can limit engagement with psychological therapies[1,2].

Clozapine and sedation

Most antipsychotics have been associated with causing sedation and among the second generation antipsychotics clozapine is reported to have the highest incidence[3]. Approximately 45% of people prescribed clozapine report sedation, hypersomnia or sleepiness, making it the most common adverse effect[1,4]. Although there are few investigative data, sedation appears to be more common in the initial weeks of treatment and tolerance is said to develop over 2–3 months[5]. In a minority of clozapine users however, sedation can be persistent and severe[1]. The mechanism behind antipsychotic-induced sedation is most likely blockade of the histamine H_1 receptor. Histamine H_1-antagonism is associated with decreased wakefulness, induced sedation and drowsiness and may have a role in regulating the sleep-wake cycle (e.g. by altering the circadian rhythm)[1]. Clozapine is a potent H_1-receptor antagonist (binding affinity, Ki=1.2nM)[1].

Treatment of clozapine-induced sedation

Although sedation is the most common adverse effect of clozapine, there are few studies investigating treatment strategies. Giving reassurance that this effect is often transient may be adequate, but this is not in fact the case for many. For those with prolonged symptoms, eliminating or reducing the dose of other medication which may cause sedation (e.g. benzodiazepines, mirtazapine or other antipsychotics) and investigating for comorbidities which are associated with tiredness (e.g. hypothyroidism, anaemia, depression or anxiety) can be fruitful. Then, the clinician should consider if the clozapine dose can be reduced (guided by plasma levels, efficacy and risk), or alter the dose to give a higher proportion in the evening. Peak plasma levels are achieved at a mean of 2.1 hours (range 0.4–4.2 hours), with a mean half life of 12 hours (range 6–26 hours)[6]. Adjusting the timing and amount of dose to the evening may help lessen sedation by reducing peak levels during the day. Although there are no formal studies investigating clozapine single dosing (usually at night), this is occasionally done in practice for those unable to tolerate a morning or lunchtime dose. If considering once-daily dosing, the healthcare team should be mindful of emerging adverse effects the following day (especially hypotension, dizziness and seizures). A controversial approach, with conflicting evidence, is to combine a CNS stimulant such as modafinil with clozapine to increase wakefulness (*Table 5.11.1*). This should be considered as a last resort because of the risk of worsening psychosis, agitation and tachycardia[7]. The only RCT focusing on clozapine and modafinil in combination failed to show any significant effect on wakefulness or fatigue[8]. There is also a single case report of modafinil increasing clozapine plasma levels and causing dizziness, tachycardia and an unsteady gait[11]. There are two cases in the literature of the successful use of methylphenidate[9].

Table 5.11.1: Stimulants investigated for clozapine-induced sedation

Author/ type of study	Number of participants	Study duration	Drug/daily dose, mg.	Outcome
Burke et al 1993 (case report)[9]	2	n/a	Case 1 = methylphenidate 30mg Case 2 = methylphenidate 5mg	Reported to be effective and well tolerated
Freudenreich et al 2009 (RCT)[8]	35	8 weeks	Modafinil up to 300mg	No significant effect on wakefulness or fatigue demonstrated (p=0.997)
Kouroumalos et al 2009 (prospective case series)[10]	10	3 months follow-up	Modafinil mean dose 110mg	All patients reported a decrease in sleep hours per day (from 11 hours to 8 hours). The improvement occurred after a week of starting modafinil and persisted to end date

Clozapine and sleep architecture

Sleep disturbances (especially insomnia) are a common feature in schizophrenia and even those who have never been medicated demonstrate altered sleep architecture compared with normal controls[12]. In schizophrenia, total sleep time and stage 4 sleep (slow-wave sleep with delta wave activity[1]) are reduced, the number of nocturnal awakenings is increased and stage 2 sleep latency is increased, equating to reduced sleep efficiency in those with schizophrenia whether or not on medication[12]. A reduction in delta waves during sleep has been associated with the severity of negative symptoms of schizophrenia[12]. Clozapine has been shown to increase total sleep time and stage 2 sleep and improve sleep efficiency[12]. Stage 4 sleep appears to be reduced in clozapine users, but rapid eye movement (REM) sleep appears not to be affected[12]. Thus, limited studies suggest that clozapine may improve sleep induction and maintenance[12], but that it does not improve delta wave activity. This is perhaps reinforced by the observation that rebound insomnia is a prominent feature when clozapine is suddenly discontinued[13].

Summary

- Approximately 45% of people prescribed clozapine report hypersomnia or sleepiness during treatment.
- Sedation appears to be more common in the initial weeks of treatment and some tolerance often develops over 2–3 months.
- For those with prolonged symptoms, review other sedating medication and investigate for any contributing comorbidities.
- Reducing the dose of clozapine or giving a higher proportion of the dose in the evening may improve daytime sedation.
- Stimulants such as modafinil combined with clozapine should only be considered as a last resort and used with extreme caution.
- Clozapine may improve sleep induction and maintenance in people with schizophrenia and sleep disturbances.

Further reading

Kane J, Sharif Z. Atypical antipsychotics: Sedation versus efficacy. *J Clin Psychiatry* 2008; **69(suppl 1):** 18–31

References

1. Kane J, Sharif Z. Atypical antipsychotics: Atypical antipsychotics: Sedation versus efficacy. *J Clin Psychiatry* 2008; **69(suppl 1):** 18–31
2. Miller D. Atypical antipsychotics: Sleep, sedation, and efficacy. *Primary Care Companion J Clin Psychiatry* 2004; **6(suppl 2):** 3–7
3. Asenjo Lobos C, Komossa K, Rummel-Kluge C, Hunger H, Schmid F, Schwarz S, Leucht S. Clozapine versus other atypical antipsychotics for schizophrenia. Cochrane Database of Systematic Reviews 2010, Issue 11. Art. No.: CD006633. DOI: 10.1002/14651858.CD006633.pub2
4. McEvoy JP, Lieberman JA, Stroup TS, Davis SM, Meltzer HY, Rosenheck RA, et al. Effectiveness of clozapine versus olanzapine, quetiapine, and risperidone in patients with chronic schizophrenia who did not respond to prior atypical antipsychotic treatment. *Am J Psychiatry* 2006; **163:** 600–10
5. Miller D. Review and management of clozapine side effects. *J Clin Psychiatry* 2000; **61(suppl 8):** 14–17
6. Clozaril specific product characteristics (SPC). Novartis. www.medicines.org.uk (accessed January 2013)
7. Provigil (modafinil) specific product characteristics (SPC). Cephalon. www.medicines.org.uk (accessed January 2013)
8. Freudenreich O, Henderson D, Macklin E, Evins E, Fan X, Cather C, et al. Modafinil for clozapine-treated schizophrenia patients: A double-blind, placebo-controlled pilot trial. *J Clin Psychiatry* 2009; **70:** 1674–80

9. Burke M, Sebastian S. Treatment of clozapine sedation. *Am J Psychiatry* 1993; **150:** 1900–01

10. Kouroumalos N, Georgila P, Marini E, Sakkras D. Modafinil's efficacy in treating clozapine-associated sedation and sleepiness in patients with schizophrenia. *J Cancer Educ* 2009; **24:** S491

11. Dequardo J. Modafinil-associated clozapine toxicity. *Am J Psychiatry* 2002; **159:** 1243–4

12. Monti J, Monti D. Sleep in schizophrenia patients and the effects of antipsychotic drugs. *Sleep Med Rev* 2004; **8:** 133–48

13. Staedt J, Stoppe G, Hajak G, Ruther E. Rebound insomnia after abrupt clozapine withdrawal. *Eur Arch Psychiatry Clin Neurosci* 1999; **246:** 79–82

5.12: Obsessive compulsive symptoms

The relationship between clozapine and worsening or developing obsessive compulsive symptoms (OCS) or obsessive compulsive disorder (OCD) is complex. Both OCS and OCD are common in schizophrenia. Between 10–64% of those with schizophrenia are reported to have OCS, while 7.8–29.8% have comorbid OCD[1, 2]. In comparison, the individual life time prevalence rate for OCD in the general population lies between 2 and 3%[3]. Some have suggested that there may be enough evidence for a special category of schizophrenia, coined as schizo-obsessive, and that the two disorders are merely different expressions of the same disease[1]. Reports however, from the last three decades have revealed higher comorbidity rates of schizophrenia and OCD than previously recognized[1, 2], and this coincides with the increasing use of the second generation antipsychotics which may be a contributing factor.

Many second generation antipsychotics (specifically olanzapine, risperidone and quetiapine[4]) have been reported to worsen or cause *de novo* OCS or OCD. Clozapine has the most reports with over 30 individual cases published. The first two cases appeared in 1992, a year after clozapine received a UK licence[5]. Since then, there have been a number of more extensive studies (*Table 5.12.1*).

It is not possible to infer the exact relationship between clozapine and OCS. The incidence of *de novo* OCS while on clozapine is reported to be between 3.5 and 28.4%[9, 10], a figure which intersects the naturally occurring incidence of comorbid schizophrenia and OCS. Some have been unable to establish any relationship[6, 14], and a small case series suggested clozapine may be beneficial in specific sub-groups of patients with OCS and schizophrenia[16], although this is disputed by others[17].

Overall, the majority of the literature tentatively suggests an increased risk of OCS and OCD associated with clozapine, which is more likely at a higher dose[10]. Reasons for a possible link between clozapine and OCS include a dopaminergic/serotoninergic imbalance, supersensitivity at 5-HT_{2C} receptors, specific neuromorphological abnormalities[18], or alterations in serotonin metabolism[19]. Case reports of successful treatment of clozapine induced OCD/OCS include lowering the dose[20], aripiprazole[21, 22, 23], sertraline[24, 25], valproic acid[26, 27], paroxetine[28], clomipramine[29] and fluvoxamine[30]. Fluvoxamine however, has been associated with a potentially toxic increase in clozapine levels so should be avoided.

Those with OCS and schizophrenia tend to have more pronounced symptoms (both positive and negative)[31], poorer social functioning, more motor symptoms[6] and a higher incidence of depression than seen in the individual illnesses[18]. Clinicians should be mindful of the link between OCD, OCS and schizophrenia and the possible increased risk incurred when starting clozapine.

Table 5.12.1: Characteristics of studies investigating clozapine causing or worsening OCS/OCD

Authors	Diagnosis	Methodology	Sample characteristics	Mean latent period before OCS reported	Outcome
Bleakley et al 2011[6]	Schizo-phrenia (86%), variety of other diagnoses	Retro-spective notes review	N=49	5–9 months	Unable to establish a relationship between clozapine and OCD Three reports (6%) of *de novo* OCS. More reports of OCS in the year before clozapine
Mukho padhaya et al 2009[7]	Schizo-phrenia/ schizo-affectice disorder	Naturalistic cross-sectional survey	N= 59	–	Unable to establish a relationship between clozapine and OCD 14 (24%) scored positively for OCD 64% had clinically meaningful OCS 50% of those with OCD were undiagnosed
Sa et al, 2009[8]	Schizo-phrenia	Cross-sectional study	N=40 on clozapine N= 20 on haloperidol	–	8 (20%) of clozapine patients had OCD vs 2 (10%) on haloperidol
Mahen-dran et al, 2007[9]	Schizo-phrenia/ schizo-affectice disorder	Cross sectional study	N=138 on clozapine (other atypical anti-psychotics were included)	5.78 months (including all atypicals investigated)	2 (3.5%) had *de novo* OCS on clozapine
Lin et al, 2006[10]	Schizo-phrenia	Cross sectional study	N=102 receiving clozapine	39.8 months	39 (38.2%) patients presented with OCS, 29 (28.4%) were considered clozapine induced. Higher plasma level of clozapine and norclozapine were associated with a higher risk of OCS
Ertugrul et al, 2005 (short report)[11]	Schizo-phrenia	Retro-spective chart review	N=50	–	10 (20%) had new onset OCS, 9 (18%) had exacerbation of preexisting OCS, 19 (38%) had OCS before clozapine of which 17 (34%) reported no change, 2 (4%) reported decrease in symptoms after clozapine initiated

Table 5.12.1: Characteristics of studies investigating clozapine causing or worsening OCS/OCD *continued*

Authors	Diagnosis	Methodology	Sample characteristics	Mean latent period before OCS reported	Outcome
De Hann et al 2004, (letter)[12]	Schizo-phrenia/ schizo-affectice disorder/ schizo-phreniform disorder	Retro-spective chart review	N=41	–	4 (9.8%) had OCD before starting clozapine and showed an improvement when clozapine started, another 4 (9.8%) developed *de novo* OCD on clozapine
De Hann et al, 1999 (short report)[13]	Schizo-phrenia, schizo-affective, schizo-phreniform, psychotic disorder	Retro-spective chart review	N= 121 (32, 26% were on clozapine)	–	7 (20.6%) patients reported an increase in obsessions after clozapine initiation, 5 had no previous obsessions
Ghaemi S et al, 1995[14]	Wide variety of diagnosis	Retro-spective chart review	N=142	–	Unable to establish a relationship between clozapine and OCD 2 (1.4%) experienced worsening OCD, no reports of *de novo* OCD due to clozapine 5 patients experienced no change in preexisting OCD after clozapine
Baker et al, 1992[15]	Schizo-phrenia	Retro-spective chart review	N=49	26.7 weeks (± 22.8 weeks)	5 (10.2%) patients experienced either *de novo* or exacerbation of OCS

– = not reported

Summary

- Obsessive compulsive symptoms (OCS) or obsessive compulsive disorder (OCD) are common in schizophrenia, even in the absence of antipsychotics.
- Screening for OCD should occur in all patients with schizophrenia.

- Many atypical antipsychotics have rare reports of *de novo* or worsening OCS/OCD. Clozapine has by far the most reports, although a direct relationship is not established.
- Emerging or worsening OCS may occur at any time of clozapine therapy and should be monitored for routinely.
- Those who develop OCS while on clozapine may respond to a lowering of the dose, or conventional OCD treatments such as an selective serotonin re-uptake inhibitor (SSRI) (not fluvoxamine) or clomipramine.

Further reading

Poyurovsky M, Weizman A, Weizman R. Obsessive-Compulsive Disorder in Schizophrenia. Clinical Characteristics and Treatment. *CNS Drugs* 2004; **18:** 989–1010

References

1. Bottas A, Cooke R, Richter M. Comorbidity and pathophysiology of obsessive-compulsive disorder in schizophrenia: Is there evidence for a schizo-obsessive subtype of schizophrenia? *J Psychiatry Neurosci* 2005; **20:** 187–93
2. Nolfe G, Milano W, Zontini G, et al. Obsessive-compulsive symptoms in schizophrenia: Their relationship with clinical features and pharmacological treatment. *J Psychiatric Practice* 2010; **16:** 235–42
3. National Institute for Health and Clinical Excellence. *Obsessive Compulsive Disorder. Clinical Guideline 31*. Available at: http://www.nice.org.uk. 2006
4. Lykouras L, Alevizos B, Michalopoulou P, et al. Obsessive-compulsive symptoms induced by atypical antipsychotics. A review of the reported cases. *Prog Neuropsychopharmacol Biol Psychiatry* 2003; **27:** 333–46
5. Patil VJ. Development of transient obsessive-compulsive symptoms during treatment with clozapine. *Am J Psychiatry* 1992; **149:** 272
6. Bleakley S, Brown D, Taylor D. Does clozapine cause or worsen OCD. An analysis and literature review. *Ther Adv Psychopharmacol* 2011; **1:** 181–8
7. Mukhopadhaya K, Krishnaiah R, Taye T, et al. Obsessive-compulsive disorder In UK clozapine-treated schizophrenia and schizoaffective disorder: a cause for clinical concern. *J Psychopharmacol* 2009; **23:** 6–13
8. Sa AR, Hounie AG, Sampaio AS, et al. Obsessive-compulsive symptoms and disorder in patients with schizophrenia treated with clozapine or haloperidol. *Compre Psychiatry* 2009; **50:** 437–42
9. Mahendran Rathi, Liew E, Subramaniam M. *De novo* emergence of obsessive-compulsive symptoms with atypical antipsychotics in Asian patients with schizophrenia or schizoaffective disorder: a retrospective, cross-sectional study. *J Clin Psychiatry* 2007; **68:** 542–5
10. Lin SK, Su SF, Pan CH. Higher plasma drug concentration in clozapine-treated schizophrenia patients with side effects of obsessive/compulsive symptoms. *Ther Drug Monit* 2006; **28:** 303–7
11. Ertugrul A, Yagcioglu E, Eni N, et al. Obsessive-compulsive symptoms in clozapine-treated

schizophrenia patients. *Psychiatry Clin Neurosci* 2005; **59:** 219–22

12. de Haan L, Oekeneva A, Van Amelsvoort T, el al. Obsessive-compulsive disorder and treatment with clozapine in 200 patients with recent-onset schizophrenia or related disorders. *Eur Psychiatry* 2004; **19:** 524
13. de Hann, Linszen D, Gorsira R. Clozapine and obsessions in patients with recent-onset schizophrenia and other psychotic disorders. *J Clin Psychiatry* 1999; **60:** 364–5
14. Ghaemia S, Zarate C, Popli A, et al. Is there a relationship between clozapine and obsessive-compulsive disorder? A retrospective chart review. *Compre Psychiatry* 1995; **36:** 267–70
15. Baker RW, Changappa KN, Baird JW, et al. Emergence of obsessive compulsive symptoms during treatment with clozapine. *J Clin Psychiatry* 1992; **53:** 439–42
16. Reznik I, Yavin I, Stryjer R, et al. Clozapine in the treatment of obsessive-compulsive symptoms in schizophrenia: a case series. *Pharmacopsychiatry* 2004; **37:** 52–6
17. McDougle CJ, Barr LC, Goodman WK, et al. Lack of efficacy of clozapine monotherapy in refractory obsessive-compulsive disorder. *Am J Psychiatry* 1995; **152:** 1812–14
18. Nolfe G, Milano W, Zontini G, et al. Obsessive-compulsive symptoms in schizophrenia: their relationship with clinical features and pharmacological treatment. *J Psychiatr Pract* 2010; **16:** 235–42
19. Ma N, Tan L-w, Wang Q, et al. Lower levels of whole blood serotonin in obsessive-compulsive disorder and in schizophrenia with obsessive-compulsive symptoms. *Psychiatry Res* 2007; **150:** 61–9
20. Aggarwal A, sharma D, Sharma RC, et al. Obsessive-compulsive symptoms following clozapine administration. *Primary Psychiatry* 2010; **17:** 58–9
21. Peters B, de Haan L. Remission of schizophrenia psychosis and strong reduction of obsessive-compulsive disorder after adding clozapine to arripiprazole. *Prog Neuropsychopharmacol Biol Psychiatry* 2009; **33:** 1576–7
22. Englisch S, Esslinger C, Inta D, et al. Clozapine-induced obsessive-compulsive syndromes improve in combination with Aripiprazole. *Clin Neuropharmacol* 2009; **32:** 227–9
23. Villari V, Frieri T, Gagiolini A. Aripiprazole-augmentation in clozapine-associated obsessive-compulsive symptoms. *J Clin Psychopharmacol* 2011; **31:** 375
24. Rahman MS, Grace JJ, Pato MT, et al. Sertraline in the treatment of clozapine-induced obsessive-compulsive behaviour. *Am J Psychiatry* 1998; **155:** 1629–30
25. Allen L, Tejera C. Treatment of clozapine-induced obsessive-compulsive symptoms with sertraline. *Am J Psychiatry* 1994; **151:** 1096–7
26. Zink M, Englisch S, Knopf U, et al. Augmentation of clozapine with valproic acid for clozapine-induced obsessive-compulsive symptoms. *Pharmacopsychiatry* 2007; **40:** 202–3
27. Canan F, Aydinoglu U, Sinani G. Valproic acid augmentation in clozapine-associated hand-washing compulsion. *Psychiatry Clin Neurosci* 2012; **66:** 460–1
28. Strous, Rael D, Patel, et al. Clozapine and paroxetine in the treatment of schizophrenia with obsessive-compulsive features. *Am J Psychiatry* 1999; **156:** 973–4
29. Biondi M, Fedele L, Arcangeli T, et al. Development of obsessive-compulsive symptoms during clozapine treatment in schizophrenia and its positive response to Clomipramine. *Psychother Psychosom* 1999; **68:** 111–12
30. Poyurovsky M, Hermesh H, Weizman A. Fluvoxamine treatment in clozapine-induced obsessive-

compulsive symptoms in schizophrenic patients. *Clin Neuropsychiatry* 1996; **19:** 305–13
31. Cunil R, Castells X, Simeon D. Relationship between obsessive-compulsive symptomology of psychosis in schizophrenia: a systematic review and meta-analysis. *J Clin Psychiatry* 2009; **70:** 70–82

6. Plasma levels

Therapeutic drug monitoring (TDM) of clozapine is a useful tool in assisting monitoring of adherence, maximising efficacy and minimising adverse effects (*Figure 6.1* shows other indications). It should always be used in conjunction with clinical observations and prescribers should avoid making decisions about dosage based solely on plasma level measurements. It is generally best to view the most recent measurement alongside previous measurements, as there is considerable intra-patient variability brought about by such factors as sampling time and changes in bio-transformation.

Clozapine levels are best performed after the initial titration stage, once the dose has been stable for at least a week[1,2]. For meaningful results, the sample should be taken as a trough level immediately before the next dose or in the morning after an evening dose (*Figure 6.2* shows advice on the timing of clozapine sampling). Routine plasma monitoring is probably not justified, but a baseline level when clozapine has reached steady state may be useful and enables comparison with any subsequent results. Although clozapine plasma levels are broadly related to daily dose[4], there are significant differences between individuals (a coefficient of variation of 53% has been suggested[5]), which appear largely due to differences in absorption and metabolism[4]. Other factors associated with influencing clozapine levels are shown in *Figure 6.3*.

Assay methods and quality control

The most common method of determining clozapine plasma levels is using high performance liquid chromatography with ultraviolet detection[4]. Full details of the assay methods have been described by Avenoso et al[8]. To ensure quality and reliability of plasma concentrations the laboratory is required to have both internal and external quality control procedures (although this may not be a legal requirement in some countries)[1]. One such international provider of an external quality assessment or clozapine TDM is HeathControl® (Cardiff Bioanalytical Services, Cardiff, UK; www.heathcontrol.com)[1,4].

Interpreting clozapine plasma levels

There is substantial literature supporting a link between clozapine plasma levels and clinical response (*Table 6.1*). The minimum clozapine level to achieve a therapeutic response in the acute stage of treatment has been suggested as between 200mcg/L and 550mcg/L[9–15]. Expert opinion and consensus statements suggest a minimum value of 350mcg/L (350ng/ml or 0.35mg/L) is associated with an increased likelihood of response[1, 15, 16]. For relapse prevention (*Table 6.2*), a slightly lower level of 200mcg/L may be appropriate[19], although there is little evidence to support this suggestion.In long-term treatment, those who demonstrate a 40% or more decrease in clozapine levels compared with that achieved during acute treatment are at a high risk of relapse and hospitalisation[19, 20].The upper therapeutic limit of clozapine plasma levels is not well defined. Limited evidence suggests increasing beyond 600–838mcg/L does not improve clinical response, but further studies are required[22]. Higher plasma levels are associated with an increasing incidence of electroencephalogram (EEG) changes and an increased risk of seizures (*Chapter 10.7*).

Figure 6.1: Indications for therapeutic drug monitoring of clozapine[1,2]

- Assessing adherence
- A poor clinical response despite adequate dosing
- Signs of toxicity or severe adverse reactions
- When a pharmacokinetic drug interaction is suspected
- When the patient is stopping or starting smoking
- Suspected genetic polymorphism (e.g. fast or slow metabolisers)
- Switching between brands (although brands show bioequivalence)[3]

Figure 6.2: When to take clozapine blood samples based on frequency of clozapine dosing

Once a day dosing

- 12 hours after the dose (usually in the morning following an evening dose)

Twice or three times a day dosing

- Immediately before the morning dose (or 12 hours after the last dose). Avoid delaying the morning dose by more than 1–2 hours

Although 12 hours after the last dose is preferred, plasma levels taken between 11 and 13 hours after the last dose are acceptable.

Figure 6.3: Factors which influence clozapine plasma levels[2,4]

Most important

- Adherence
- Timing of sample (less significant for the norclozapine level)
- Dose
- Pharmacokinetic drug interactions
- Smoking status

May be clinically significant

- Gender (females metabolise clozapine more slowly)
- Age (younger patients demonstrate faster metabolism)
- Body weight (slightly higher doses are needed in heavier people)
- Gastrointestinal hypomotility (resulting in delayed absorption)
- Caffeine intake (may increase clozapine plasma levels via competitive inhibition of CYP 1A2)
- Genetic factors (fast or slow metabolisers)
- Ethnicity (Asian patients may show higher levels than Caucasians)[6]
- Respiratory infections (case reports suggest levels may be increased)[7]

Table 6.1: Relationship between plasma clozapine level and acute therapeutic response

Author, year	n	Duration	Dose or level achieved	Conclusion (response rate determined as 20% reduction in BPRS, unless otherwise stated)
Llorca et al, 2002[9]	37	18 weeks	Mean dose at endpoint 486.5mg/day (range 200–800mg/day)	Response rate was defined as 20% reduction in PANSS. A plasma threshold of 550mcg/L was associated with an improved clinical response. The dosing schedules may in part account for the higher plasma threshold. Dose was either given as a single dose at 8.00pm, or two divided doses at 6.00pm and 8.00pm
Spina et al, 2000[10]	45	12 weeks	Mean dose at endpoint was 309mg/day (range 200–500mg/day)	Mean plasma clozapine concentration was higher in responders than non-responders (P<0.01), but norclozapine levels did not differ significantly. A cut-off of 350mcg/L is suggested as a target for response
Van der Zwagg et al, 1996[11]	56	12 weeks	Three study groups based on clozapine level: 1. Low, 50–150mcg/L 2. Medium, 200–300mcg/L 3. High, 350–450mcg/L	Response rates were: 1. Low group, 20% response 2. Medium, 61% response 3. High, 60% response. Both medium and high plasma level groups showed greater improvement than the low level group (p=0.003)
Kronig et al, 1995[12]	45	6 weeks	Mean daily dose at endpoint was 483.9mg/day (±55.7mg)	A threshold of 350mg/L was associated with treatment response
Potkin et al, 1994[13]	58	12 weeks	Fixed dose at 400mg/day	A clozapine blood concentration of 420mg/L or higher was associated with increased chance of response. At week 12, 73% of participants above 420mg/L responded, compared with 29% responding below 420mg/L
Hasegawa et al, 1993[14]	59	6 months	Mean daily dose at endpoint in responders was 475.9mg (±195.6mg)	A clozapine concentration of 370mcg/L was determined as the minimum required for optimal response. Above 370mcg/L, 73% of participants responded, below 370mcg/L, 39% responded
Perry et al, 1991[15]	29	4 weeks	Mean dose was 384mg (±42 mg)	A clozapine plasma level of at least 350mcg/L gave a response rate of 64%, while under 350mcg/L the response rate was 22%. A cut-off clozapine concentration of 350mcg/L is suggested as the minimum effective target level

BPRS = Brief Psychiatric Rating Scale; PANSS = Positive and Negative Syndrome Scale.
Note: 1mcg/L = 1ng/ml = 0.001mg/L

Table 6.2: Relationship between plasma clozapine level and relapse prevention			
Author, year	n	Duration	Conclusion Note: 1mcg/L = 1ng/ml = 0.001mg/L
Stieffenhofer et al, 2011[18]	23	21 months	Plasma levels below the target value of 350mcg/L were associated with an 11 times higher risk of hospitalisation
Xiang et al, 2006[19]	102	1 year	33/69 relapsed and an inverse correlation between increasing BPRS and clozapine levels was identified. Relapses and non-relapses were separated by a threshold of at least 200mcg/L. A reduction of 40% of plasma levels from those achieved during acute treatment was associated with relapse
Gaertner et al, 2001[20]	23	Up to 5 years follow-up	A plasma clozapine level decrease of more than 40% from baseline was associated with an increased risk of relapse (risk ratio of 6, 95% CI 2–9, p=0.003)
Miller, 1994[21]	29	2.4 years	At endpoint, 58% of participants were classified as responders and 5/7 non-responders at week 6 responded if their clozapine plasma concentration increased above 350mg/L

Many other non-neurological adverse effects are also thought to be dose or plasma level-related (e.g. sedation, metabolic changes, hypomotility, hypersalivation) and require close monitoring in those with an increasing plasma level. Defining an upper limit for clozapine levels may prevent potentially worthwhile increases in those who tolerate clozapine well. A prophylactic anticonvulsant (e.g. lamotrigine or valproate) should be considered in those whose levels are 600mcg/L or higher. In any case, prescribers should avoid increasing levels beyond 1000mcg/L (*Table 6.3* presents advice on interpreting levels). The target plasma clozapine levels in the under 18s or over 65s are less well defined, but they are generally considered the same as adult ranges[23, 24].

Norclozapine levels

Norclozapine (N-desmethylclozapine), one of the main metabolites of clozapine, is often reported alongside clozapine plasma levels. Although there are limited data, it is considered to be at least partially active and potentially responsible for some of clozapine's unique efficacy[26]. It has a longer plasma half-life than clozapine, so is less affected by daily fluctuations in levels and is not dependent on a trough sampling time[17]. On average, the clozapine to norclozapine ratio is suggested as 1.32 across all dose ranges. Thus, at a clozapine plasma level of 350mcg/L, the average norclozapine level would be 265mcg/L (0.27mg/L)[27]. Clozapine metabolism (via cytochrome P450 1A2) may, however, become saturated as the clozapine to norclozapine ratio appears to increase at higher plasma levels (*Table 6.4*)[17]. A similar reduction in the clozapine to norclozapine ratio has been shown when fluvoxamine (a potent cytochrome P450 1A2 inhibitor) is added to clozapine, which also supports a potential saturation of the metabolising enzyme[28].

Table 6.3: Summary of clozapine plasma level interpretation (adapted with kind permission)[25]

*Trough clozapine level (12 hours post dose) mcg/L (1mcg/L = 1ng/ml = 0.001mg/L)	Clinical response	Comment
<10mcg/L or not detected	Any	Clozapine unlikely to have been taken for at least a week unless in the very early initiation stage
<350mcg/L	Good	Continue current dose, repeat levels annually or sooner if response deteriorates, or adverse reactions become troublesome
	Poor or incomplete	If poor adherence is suspected, consider education, supervised consumption, reminder cards, compliance aids or using clozapine liquid or oral disintegrating tablets (if available). If no improvement, consider a cautious increase in clozapine dose, monitoring response and tolerability. Consider repeating the assay after one week on the new dose
350–600mcg/L (target range)[1, 16]	Good	Continue current dose, review regularly for continuing response and tolerability. Consider repeating levels annually
	Poor or incomplete	If clozapine has continued for at least 3–6 months and still incomplete response, consider augmentation with another suitable psychotropic
601–999mcg/L	Good with no features of toxicity	Consider a cautious dose reduction, weighing against response, risk and tolerability. If considered essential to maintain at current dose, consider using a prophylactic anticonvulsant to protect against seizures (usually lamotrigine or valproate). Monitor closely for tolerability and response
	Poor, incomplete or features of toxicity	Consider a cautious dose reduction to bring levels under 600mcg/L, weighing against response, risk and tolerability. Repeat the assay once stabilised on a new dose
>1000mcg/L (the upper limit is not well defined)	Any	Review urgently. Consider a dose reduction to bring levels down below 1000mcg/L and ideally below 600mcg/L, weighing against risk, response and tolerability. If clinical signs of toxicity (severe sedation, delirium, falls, seizures), consider withholding clozapine for 24 hours and reintroducing at a lower dose. Consider initiating an anticonvulsant to protect against seizures. Repeat levels once the lower dose is stabilised

* Before acting on a result, clinicians are reminded to confirm the plasma sample was taken as a trough level

Table 6.4: Median clozapine to norclozapine levels and ratios (n=102,593)[17]

Clozapine level 1mcg/L = 1ng/ml = 0.001mg/L	Median clozapine to norclozapine ratio	Norclozapine level
<350mcg/L	1.25	<280mcg/L
350–600mcg/L	1.55	280–387mcg/L
601–1000mcg/L	1.78	343–562mcg/L
>1000mcg/L	2.08	>481mcg/L

Poor or non-adherence

Undetectable clozapine plasma levels clearly indicate non-adherence over at least the preceding week. The healthcare team should search for and remove the unused clozapine tablets and consider re-titrating the dose if appropriate. Partial adherence will result in unpredictable plasma levels, which are difficult to interpret and negate the benefit of TDM. Sporadic adherence with clozapine is associated with a sudden-onset psychosis and cholinergic rebound symptoms, a syndrome which will need to be highlighted to the patient, family and carers (*Chapter 4*). Even when a result is returned within the proposed target range for clozapine, this simply indicates that the drug has been taken consistently over at least the last few days. In suspected poor adherence, repeating plasma levels at irregular intervals may be useful to detect a trend in results.

Summary

- Measuring plasma clozapine levels is a useful adjunct when used in conjunction with clinical observations.
- Clozapine plasma levels are generally best performed after the initial titration stage, once the dose has been stable for at least a week.
- For accurate levels, the sample should be taken as a trough level, for example immediately before the next dose or in the morning after an evening dose (around 12 hours post dose).
- A clozapine plasma level of 350mcg/l to 600mcg/L is broadly associated with a good clinical response and may minimise toxic effects[1, 16].
- Consider a prophylactic anticonvulsant in those whose levels are 600mcg/L or higher.
- The upper limit to the clozapine plasma level is not well defined, but levels above 1000mcg/L should be avoided.

Further reading and resources

Remmington G, Agid O, Foussias G, Ferguson L, McDonald K, Powell V. Clozapine and therapeutic drug monitoring: is there sufficient evidence for an upper threshold? *Psychopharmacology* 2013; **225:** 505–18.

KingsPath, from Kings College Hospital. One of the UK's leading providers of clozapine plasma monitoring. Available at: http://kingspath.co.uk

References

1. Hiemke C, Baumann P, Bergemann N, Conca A, Dietmaier O, Egberts K, et al. AGNP consensus guidelines for therapeutic drug monitoring in psychiatry: update 2011. *Pharmacopsychiatry* 2011; **44:** 195–235
2. Greenwood-Smith C, Lubman D, Castle D. Serum clozapine levels: a review of their clinical utility. *J Psychopharmacol* 2003; **17:** 234–8
3. Couchman L, Morgan P, Spencer E, Johnston A, Flanagan R. Plasma clozapine and norclozapine in patients prescribed different brands of clozapine (Clozaril, Denzapine, and Zaponex). *Ther Drug Monit* 2010; **32:** 624–7
4. Couchman L, Morgan P, Spencer E, Flanagan R. Plasma clozapine, norclozapine, and the clozapine: norclozapine ratio in relation to prescribed dose and other factors: Data from a therapeutic drug monitoring service 1993–2007. *Ther Drug Monit* 2010; **32:** 438–47
5. Kurz M, Hummer M, Kemmler G, Kurzthaler I, Saria A, Fleischhacker W. Long-term pharmacokinetics of clozapine. *Br J Psychiatry* 1998; **173:** 341–4
6. Ng C, Chong S, Lambert T, Fan A, Hackett P, Mahendran R, Subramaniam M, Schweitzer I. An inter-ethnic comparison study of clozapine dosage, clinical response and plasma levels. *Int Clin Psychopharmacol* 2005; **20:** 163–8
7. De Leon J, Diaz F. Serious respiratory infections can increase clozapine levels and contribute to side effects: a case report. *Prog Neuropsychopharmacol Biol Psychiatry* 2003; **27:** 1059–63
8. Avenoso A, Facciolà G, Campo G, Fazio A, Spina E. Determination of clozapine, desmethylclozapine and clozapine n-oxide in human plasma by reversed-phase high performance liquid chromatography with ultraviolet detection. *J Chromatogr B Biomed Sci Appl* 1998; **714:** 299–308
9. Llorca PM, Lancon C, Disdier B, Farisse J, Sapin C, Auquier P. Effectiveness of clozapine in neuroleptic-resistant schizophrenia: clinical response and plasma concentrations. *J Psychiatry Neurosci* 2002; **27:** 30–7
10. Spina E, Avenoso A, Facciolà G, Scordo M, Ancione M, Madia A, et al. Relationship between plasma concentrations of clozapine and norclozapine and therapeutic response in patients with schizophrenia resistant to conventional neuroleptics. *Psychopharmacology* 2000; **148:** 83–9
11. VanderZwaag C, McGee M, McEvoy J, Freudenreich O, Wilson W, Cooper T. Response of patients with treatment-refractory schizophrenia to clozapine within three serum level ranges. *Am J Psychiatry* 1996; **153:** 1579–84
12. Kronig M, Munne R, Szymanski S, Safferman A, Pollack S, Cooper T, et al. Plasma clozapine levels and clinical response for treatment-refractory schizophrenia patients. *Am J Psychiatry* 1995; **2:** 179–82
13. Potkin S, Bera R, Gulasekaram B, Costa J, Hayes S, Jin Y, et al. Plasma clozapine concentrations predict clinical response in treatment-resistant schizophrenia. *J Clin Psychiatry* 1994; **55(suppl B):** 133–6
14. Hasegawa M, Gutierrez-Esteinou R, Way M, Meltzer H. Relationship between clinical efficacy and

clozapine concentrations in plasma in schizophrenia: effect of smoking. *J Clin Psychopharmacol* 1993; **13:** 383–90

15. Perry P, Miller D, Arndt S, Cadoret R. Clozapine and norclozapine plasma concentrations and clinical response of treatment-refractory schizophrenia patients. *Am J Psychiatry* 1991; **148:** 231–5.
16. Taylor D, Paton C, Kapur S. *The Maudsley Prescribing guidelines.* 11th edn: Oxford: Wiley-Blackwell: 2012
17. Couchman L, Morgan P, Spencer E, Flanagan R. Plasma clozapine, norclozapine, and the clozapine:norclozapine ratio in relation to prescribed dose and other factors: Data from a therapeutic drug monitoring service, 1993–2007. *Ther Drug Monit* 2010; **32:** 438–47
18. Stieffenhofer V, Saglam H, Schmidtmann I, Silver H, Hiemke C, Konrad A. Clozapine plasma level monitoring for prediction of rehospitalisation schizophrenia outpatients. *Pharmacopsychiatry* 2011; **44:** 55–9
19. Xiang Y, Zhang Z, Weng Y, Zhai Y, Li W, Cai Z, et al. Serum concentrations of clozapine and norclozapine in the prediction of relapse of patients with schizophrenia. *Schizophr Res* 2006; **83:** 201–10
20. Gaertner I, Gaertner H, Vonthein R, Dietz K. Therapeutic drug monitoring of clozapine in relapse prevention: A five-year prospective study. *J Clin Psychopharmacol* 2001; **21:** 305–10
21. Miller D, Fleming F, Holman T, Perry P. Plasma clozapine concentrations as a predictor of clinical response: A follow-up study. *J Clin Psychiatry* 1994; **55(suppl B):** 117–121
22. Remmington G, Agid O, Foussias G, Ferguson L, McDonald K, Powell V. Clozapine and therapeutic drug monitoring: is there sufficient evidence for an upper threshold? *Psychopharmacology* 2013; **225:** 505–18
23. Couchman L, Bowskill S, Handley S, Patel M, Flanagan R. Plasma clozapine and norclozapine in relation to prescribed dose and other factors in patients aged <18 years: data from a therapeutic drug monitoring service, 1994–2010. *Early Interv Psychiatry* 2013; **7:** 122–30
24. Bowskill S, Couchman L, MacCabe J, Flanagan R. Plasma clozapine and norclozapine in relation to prescribed dose and other factors in patients aged 65 years and over: data from a therapeutic drug monitoring service, 1996–2010. *Hum Psychopharmacol* 2012; **27:** 277–83
25. Flanagan R. A practical approach to clozapine therapeutic drug monitoring. *College of Mental Health Pharmacy Bull,* June 2010. Available at www.cmhp.org.uk
26. Mendoza M, Lindenmayer J. N-Desmethylclozapine: is there evidence for its antipsychotic potential? *Clin Neuropharmacol* 2009; **32:** 154–7
27. Rostami-Hodjegan A, Amin A, Spencer E, Lennard M, Tucker G, Flannagan R. Influence of dose, cigarette smoking, age, sex and metabolic activity on plasma clozapine concentrations: A predictive model and nomograms to aid clozapine dose adjustments and to assess compliance in individual patients. *J Clin Psychopharmacol* 2004; **24:** 70–8
28. Wang C, Zang Z, Li W, Zhai Y, Cai Z, Weng Y, et al. The differential effects of steady-state fluvoxamine on the pharmacokinetics of olanzapine and clozapine in healthy volunteers. *J Clin Pharmacol* 2004; **44:** 785–92

7. Pharmacogenetic testing

An intriguing recent development across CNS disorders is the concept of personalised prescribing or tailoring the drug treatment to the individual. This attempts to identify genetic markers to help predict response to drug treatment or to predict troublesome adverse effects. Clozapine has been the subject of a few emerging tests which are outlined in brief below. A complication when reviewing these tests is a lack of readily available published data. As this is a commercially sensitive issue, few companies publish complete details of the exact genes or variations in genes identified in the tests.

Predicting response to clozapine: the LGC predict test

Genetic variation in 5-HT_{2a} receptors has been shown to be one factor in predicting response to clozapine[1]. Other receptor polymorphisms are also involved and in 2000, Arranz et al at the Institute of Psychiatry London, published their results investigating 19 polymorphisms across nine genes. Two hundred patients with schizophrenia treated with clozapine were investigated, and a combination of six polymorphisms showed the strongest association of response to clozapine (5-HT2a102-T/C and His452Tyr, 5-HT2c-330-GT/-244-CT and Cys23Ser, 5-HTTLPR, H2-1018-G/A). This gave a prediction level of 76.86% with a sensitivity of 95%[2]. Unfortunately, the findings were not replicated in a German sample of 163 patients on clozapine[3], but sample differences (e.g. ethnic origin and duration of treatment) may have accounted for the lack of replication[4]. Based on the Arranz study (and presumably further unpublished work), the UK company, LGC, developed and launched a clozapine predictive test in 2005[5]. This test collected cheek cells via a buccal swab and gave a predictive percentage chance of responding to clozapine. Unfortunately, due to sporadic requests for the test and subsequent difficulties in maintaining competency and accreditation, the test was suspended in April 2010, but the company remain committed to re-launching the test should demand increase[6].

Predicting agranulocytosis: Pgxpredict: clozapine test

A genetic test to predict clozapine-induced agranulocytosis was developed by PGxHealth (a division of Clinical Data, a diagnostic company in the US). The test was called PGxPredict: Clozapine but, unfortunately, is no longer available or advertised[7]. Two of the three genes described in this test were from the HLA complex, the other three genes remain unpublished and may provide targets for future research[7].

Cytochrome P450 testing

Clozapine is primarily metabolised by the cytochrome P450 enzyme 1A2, with a variety of other metabolic pathways (CYP 2D6, 3A4, 2C9/19 and UGT 1A3/4) playing a minor role (*Chapter 8*). Cytochromes 1A2, 2D6 and 2C19 are subject to much genetic polymorphism which can unpredictably affect clozapine response and tolerability. Commercially available pharmacogenetic testing is available for cytochromes 1A2, 2D6, 2C9 and 2C19[8]. The American company, Genelex®, provide the widest range of cytochrome genotyping testing[8], of which the 1A2 test is probably the most beneficial in regards to predicting clozapine metabolism. Two polymorphisms in the CYP1A2*1 wild-type allele have been identified and are targets for the Genelex 1A2 test. The CYP1A2*1C allele is the result of a single point mutation (-3860 G>A) and is associated with decreased (or a poor metaboliser) activity. The CYP1A2*1F allele is another single point mutation (-163 C>A) and is associated with increased (or a fast metaboliser) activity, particularly in smokers[9]. While this test does not rule out all known mutations in CYP1A2, it goes part of the way to explaining why individual response and tolerability to clozapine vary considerably.

Roche Molecular Diagnostics® have available the AmpliChip® CYP450 Test[10]. This provides an extensive analysis of CYP2D6 and 2C19 genetic polymorphisms (testing for 29 known polymorphisms in the CYP2D6 gene and two major polymorphisms in the CYP2C19 gene)[10]. Although 2D6 is a minor metabolic pathway for clozapine, this test may be useful for those with a normal 1A2 activity, but still show an abnormal response or tolerability to clozapine.

Metabolic syndrome testing

The American biomedical company Genomas® are developing a metabolic risk test for olanzapine, risperidone and quetiapine (known as the PIMS PhyzioType System®)[11]. This test uses a variety of DNA markers coupled with a biostatistical algorithm to predict an individual's risk for metabolic syndrome.

Summary

- Pharmacogenetic testing provides an intriguing opportunity to tailor clozapine dosing and monitoring to the individual patient based on their genetic profile.
- Cytochrome P450 genotyping is the most widely available test and may help identify poor or fast clozapine metabolisers.

Web addresses for further information

LGC predict test:	http://www.lgc.co.uk
Genelex CYP1A2 gentotyping	http://www.healthanddna.com/

Roche AmpliChip http://www.roche.com
PIMS PhyzioType System: http://www.genomas.net

Further reading

Leon J. Pharmacogenomics: The promise of personalized medicine for CNS disorders. *Neuropsychopharmacology* 2008; **34:** 159–72

References

1. Arranz MJ, Munro J, Sham P et al. Meta-analysis of studies on genetic variation in 5-HT2a receptors and clozapine response. *Schizophr Res* 1998; **32:** 93–9
2. Arranz M, Munro J, Birkett J, Bolonna A, Mancama D, Sodhi M, et al. Pharmacogenetic prediction of clozapine response. *Lancet* 2000; **355:** 1615–6
3. Schumacher J, Schulze T, Weinker T, Rietschel M, Nöthen M Pharmacogentics of clozapine response. *Lancet* 2000; **356:** 506–7
4. Arranz M, Munro J, Osborne S, Collier D, Kerwin R Difficulties in replication of results. *Lancet* 2000; **356:** 1359–60
5. LGC. http://www.lgc.co.uk (accessed July 2012)
6. Barallon R. LGC predict test. 29 May 2012
7. Leon J. Pharmacogenomics: The promise of personalized medicine for CNS disorders. *Neuropsychopharmacology* 2008; **34:** 159–72
8. Genelex. Cytochrome genotyping. Available at: http://www.healthanddna.com (accessed July 2012)
9. Doherty D. Genelex 1A2 genotyping. 26 June 2012
10. Roche Molecular Diagnostics. AmpliChip. Available at: http://www.roche.com (accessed July 2012)
11. Genomas. PIMS PhyzioType System. Available at: http://www.genomas.net (accessed July 2012)

8. Drug interactions

Predicting clozapine interactions can be complex and unpredictable, but using a few simple questions can help highlight potential problems:

- Do any drugs being added to clozapine cause similar side-effects?
- Does the potential combination of drugs (or other substances) affect the way clozapine is handled by the body?
- Does the patient's physical state or comorbidities increase the risks associated with prescribing clozapine?

Do any drugs being added to clozapine cause similar side-effects? (pharmacodynamic interaction)

Clozapine has a complex neurotransmitter profile, which in part explains its many adverse reactions. Before starting clozapine or adding another medication to clozapine, clinicians should consider if additive side-effects may be a problem. Many other drugs added to clozapine have potential pharmacodynamic interactions. These include:

- Sedative drugs, increasing the risk of clozapine-induced sedation
- Antihypertensive drugs, adding to the risk of postural hypotension and falls
- Pro-convulsant drugs, adding to the risk of clozapine-induced seizures.

While there are few absolute contraindications, clinicians should be mindful of additive side-effects and may wish to instigate additional monitoring. *Table 8.1* considers common pharmacodynamic interactions.

Does the potential combination of drugs (or substances) affect the way clozapine is handled by the body? (pharmacokinetic interaction)

Most drugs given orally undergo various processes in the body. This includes absorption of the drug from the gut into the blood stream, distribution of the drug around the body into various tissues, metabolism (predominantly by the liver) to enable the drug to be removed by the body and elimination, which describes the final exit of the drug from the body (usually by the kidneys). This process is commonly known as ADME (absorption, distribution, metabolism and elimination). At any point in the bio-transformation of clozapine by the body, other drugs can affect the process.

The most startling pharmacokinetic interactions are often caused by drugs which are either enzyme inhibitors or enzyme inducers. Enzyme inhibition is a rapid process with increased adverse effects and risk of toxicity occurring over 2–3 days. Enzyme induction is a more gradual process occurring between 1–3 weeks[1]. An example of a commonly quoted enzyme inhibitor of clozapine is fluvoxamine.

Table 8.1: Common pharmacodynamic interactions to consider with clozapine (drugs in CAPITALS are particularly hazardous and should be avoided)[1,2,3]

Potential additive side-effects	Drug or class
Increased risk of neutropenia/ aganulocytosis	CARBAMAZEPINE CARBIMAZOLE CHLORAMPHENICOL CYTOTOXICS (*Chapter 9*) LONG-ACTING DEPOT ANTIPSYCHOTCS PENICILLAMINE PHENYLBUTAZONE Rarely other antipsychotics SULPHONAMIDES (e.g. co-trimoxazole)
Increased sedation	Alcohol Antihistamines Benzodiazepines Mirtazapine Opioid analgesics Other antipsychotics Trazodone Tricyclic antidepressants
Increased risk of anticholinergic side-effects (e.g. constipation, urinary retention, blurred vision, confusion)	Anticholinergic drugs (procyclidine, hyoscine, etc) Other antipsychotics Tricyclic antidepressants
Increased risk of constipation (other than anticholinergics)	LOPERAMIDE Opioid analgesics
Decreased blood pressure or falls	ACE inhibitors Alcohol Antihypertensives Other antipsychotics Tricyclic antidepressants
Increased risk of seizures	Other antipsychotics Sudden benzodiazepine withdrawal Tricyclic antidepressants
Increased weight gain/ metabolic changes	Lithium Mirtazapine Otherantipsychotics Tricyclic antidepressants Valproate

Fluvoxamine has been shown to dramatically increase clozapine levels by up to 10-fold[1], having the potential to cause life-threatening side-effects. The mechanism underpinning this dramatic interaction is that fluvoxamine is a potent inhibitor of the liver P450 isoenzyme CYP1A2. This enzyme is the main metabolic pathway for clozapine conversion to norclozapine, so any drug or substance affecting CYP1A2 can significantly alter clozapine levels[5]. Clozapine is also metabolised by a variety of other metabolic pathways (CYP 2D6, 3A4, 2C9/19, UGT 1A3/4 and a flavin monooxygenase)[2,6]. These are less important routes for clozapine metabolism, so are less likely to cause significant interactions, but considering the potential toxicity of clozapine they should also be considered. *Table 8.2* shows the main metabolic pathways of clozapine and drugs and substances which can affect clozapine levels. *Table 8.3* displays the full pharmacokinetic properties of clozapine at steady state in adults and *Table 8.4* shows the metabolic processes of clozapine.

Does the patient's physical state or comorbidities increase the risks associated with prescribing clozapine?

Impaired physical health can increase the risks associated with prescribing clozapine, or affect the way clozapine is altered by the body. For example, clozapine, particularly at high doses or during a fast dose titration, may cause seizures which can destabilise a patient with epilepsy. Elderly patients are particularly prone to the hypotensive, anticholinergic and falls risk with clozapine. Patients with hepatic impairment may accumulate clozapine and the sedative and constipating effects can increase the risk of hepatic encephalopathy. *Table 8.5* considers how physical comorbidities can increase the risks associated with prescribing clozapine. *Chapter 10* contains an in-depth discussion on prescribing clozapine in special patient populations.

Table 8.2: Drugs and substances which can affect the metabolic pathways of clozapine (drugs in CAPITALS are particularly hazardous and should be avoided)[1,2,3]

Metabolising enzymes					
P450 CYP1A2 # (major pathway, likely to cause clinically significant interactions)		P450 CYP2D6 # (minor pathways, occasional clinical significance)		P450 CYP3A4 (minor pathways, occasional clinical significance)	
Inhibitor (likely to increase clozapine levels)	Inducer (likely to reduce clozapine levels)	Inhibitor (may increase clozapine levels)	Inducer (may reduce clozapine levels)	Inhibitor (may increase clozapine levels)	Inducer (may reduce clozapine levels)
Caffeine (n=22, 14–47%↑) Ciprofloxacin (n=10, 29–31%↑) Disulfiram* Norfloxacin* FLUVOXAMINE (multiple studies, up to 10-fold elevations in clozapine levels) Oral contraceptive (norethisterone/ ehinylestradiol) n=2, ?↑) significance unclear.	Omeprazole (n=15, up to 45%↓) Phenobarbital (n=8, 35%↓) Phenytoin (n=3, 65–85%↓) Primidone* RIFAMPICIN (n=2, up to 600%↓) Tipranavir* Tobacco smoke (multiple studies, 50–72%↓)	Fluoxetine (multiple studies, 30–75%↑) Paroxetine (multiple studies, 0–57%↑) Sertraline — probably dose dependent. (n=21,0–52%↑) Ritonavir*	Nil of note	Cimetidine (n=2, up to 60%↑) Clarithromycin* Erythromycin (n=14, 0%↑ — toxicity, reported) Oral contraceptive (norethisterone/ ehinylestradiol) n=2, ?↑) significance unclear. Ritonavir* Telithromycin*	CARBAMAZE-PINE (multiple studies, 50%↓) RIFAMPICIN (n=2, up to 600%↓)

Note: There are no significant clozapine interactions reported solely by the CYP 2C9/19, UGT or FMO metabolic routes. # = subject to genetic polymorphism; n = the number of case reports on the interaction; % = the percentage change in clozapine levels reported; * = no current literature available on the interaction; ? = unknown percentage change in clozapine levels

It would be almost impossible to avoid all potentially interacting drugs, substances or disease states concurrently with clozapine. However, clinicians should be aware of the potential interactions, inform the patient and monitor closely for any increased adverse reactions. Altering the dose of clozapine or choosing a drug which is less likely to interact may also be an option.

It is also important to remember that drug interactions are notoriously poorly studied with most only reported in case series or case reports. Confusingly, there are reports of drugs with established interactions, having no effect at all and being well tolerated[1]. This unpredictability suggests that patient variability is considerable and no 'one size fits all'.

Table 8.3: The pharmacokinetic properties of oral clozapine at steady state in adults[3, 12]

Absorption	First pass metabolism	Peak plasma levels	Volume of distribution	Plasma protein binding	Half-life	Metabolising enzymes	Main metabolites	Excretion
90–95% not influenced by food	Moderate Overall bioavailability 50–60%	0.4–4.2 hours (mean 2.1 hours)	1.6 L/kg	Clozapine 95% Norclozapine 90% Clozapine-N-oxide 75%	Biphasic Single dose 8 hours, Steady state mean 14.2 hours	Major CYP1A2 Minor CYP 2D6, CYP 3A4, CYP 2C9/19 UGT 1A3/4	Desmethyl-clozapine or norclozapine (active) clozapine-N-oxide (inactive)	50% in the urine 30% in the faeces

Cytochrome genetic polymorphism

One factor which contributes to the unpredictability of clozapine interactions is that the P450 enzymes are subject to much genetic polymorphism. With clozapine metabolism, the P450 isoenzymes CYP 1A2, 2D6 and 2C19 are subject to polymorphism. For example, 12% of the white population are thought to be poor

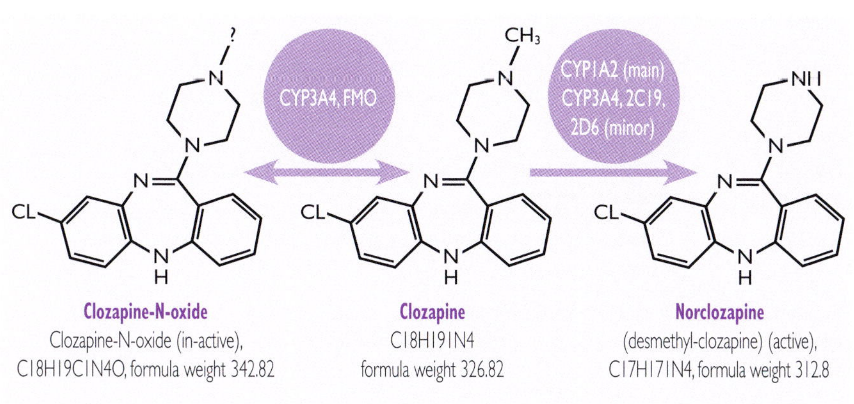

Figure 8.1: The main metabolic processes of clozapine[11, 12] (the ration of clozapine:norclozapine: clozapine-N-oxide is 1:1:2)

metabolisers (they are less efficient at metabolising clozapine) at CYP 1A2, while 3–10% of the white population are poor metabolisers at CYP 2D6[7,8]. In addition, up to 29% of North Africans and those from the Middle East are ultra fast metabolisers at CYP 2D6[8]. Cytochrome P450 3A4 shows little polymorphism[2]. Pharmacogenetic tests for CYP polymorphisms are becoming commercially available and can help identify those for whom extra monitoring is advocated (*Chapter* 7).

Table 8.4: Physical states or comorbidities which increase the risks associated with prescribing clozapine[2,3,4]

	Potential risk
Cardiovascular disease	Increased tachycardia, postural hypotension, rare reports of cardiomyopathy or myocarditis. Clozapine commonly causes weight gain, hypertension and hyperlipidaemia which may increase cardiovascular risk. Contraindicated in severe cardiac disorders
Dementia	Clozapine's anticholinergic properties may reduce the effectiveness of the acetylcholinesterase inhibitors used in Alzheimer's disease. In line with other antipsychotics, clozapine may increase the risk of cerebral vascular accidents and reduce life expectancy when used in dementia
Diabetes mellitus	May cause or worsen diabetes
Epilepsy	Increased risk of seizures (particularly at high doses or a fast dose titration). Contraindicated in uncontrolled epilepsy
Glaucoma (narrow angled)	Clozapine's anticholinergic properties have the potential to cause or worsen glaucoma
Hepatic impairment	Potential accumulation of clozapine and increased risk of hepatic encephalopathy. Contraindicated in severe hepatic impairment
Impaired bone marrow function	Contraindicated because of the increased risk of blood disorders
Old age	Clozapine may accumulate due to reduce hepatic and renal function. Use lower doses and increase slowly in the elderly. More sensitive to anticholinergic and postural hypotensive side-effects. May increase the risk of falls
Prostatic enlargement	Clozapine's anticholinergic properties have the potential to cause or worsen prostatic enlargement
Renal impairment	Contraindicated in severe renal disease, nocturnal enuresis and urinary retention commonly reported
Respiratory infections	Potential increased risk from clozapine-induced hypersalivation. Also, intriguingly, the infection itself may increase clozapine levels by CYP 1A2 inhibition[9]

Non-prescribed drugs to consider

Smoking

Tobacco smoke contains polycyclic aromatic hydrocarbons which are potent inducers of CYP 1A2. Smokers on clozapine consistently show up to 50% lower plasma levels than non-smokers[1]. Smoking as few as 7–12 cigarettes per day may be sufficient to cause the maximum enzyme induction[1]. Consequently, giving up smoking can cause an increase in clozapine levels between 50 and 72%, which can lead to severe adverse effects such as seizures (nicotine replacement or chewing tobacco does not ameliorate the interaction)[10]. The interaction usually occurs gradually between two and four weeks and can be especially difficult to predict in those sporadically stopping and starting smoking. Clinicians should monitor clozapine levels before stopping smoking, reduce the dose gradually by approximately 25% and recheck levels four weeks after stopping smoking[4]. Further dose adjustments should be made in light of any emerging clozapine side-effects or toxicity. Smoking cannabis cut with tobacco is likely to cause a similar interaction.

Caffeine

Excessive caffeine consumption (i.e. above 250mg per day, or 4–5 cups of coffee per day) can cause psychotropic effects such as restlessness, excitement, insomnia and possibly worsens psychosis[4]. In addition, it has been suggested that clozapine and caffeine compete for the same metabolic pathway (CYP 1A2) which may result in an increase in clozapine levels. The effect is subject to much patient variability but increased clozapine levels between 14 and 47% have been reported[1]. In those on a stable clozapine dose where caffeine intake remains predictable, this is unlikely to be a problem but, for patients taking high caffeine preparations (found in some soft drinks and herbal products), extra monitoring for adverse effects is recommended.

Cocaine

A single study in eight cocaine addicts suggested clozapine dramatically increased cocaine levels by up to 67%, depending on the clozapine dose. A reduction in the cocaine 'high' was also noted[1,2]. Considering the potential cardiac adverse effects of both cocaine and clozapine, combining them is highly risky.

Summary

- Clozapine has the potential to cause multiple interactions. These can be grouped as pharmacodynamic or pharmacokinetic interactions, or a physical comorbidity which increases the risks of prescribing clozapine.
- Predicting potential interactions is complex and subject to patient variations.
- Genetic polymorphism of the metabolising CYP enzymes may account for part of this unpredictability.

- Ideally, interacting drugs should be avoided where possible.
- Few interactions however are an absolute contraindication, but many require additional monitoring or adjustment of the clozapine dose.

Further reading

Baxter K. *Stockley's Drug Interactions.* 9th edn. London: Pharmaceutical Press: 2010

Sandson N, Cozza K, Armstrong S, Eckermann G, Fischer B, Phillips B.Med-Psych Drug interaction update. Clozapine case series. *Psychosomatics* 2007; **48:** 170–5

References

1. Baxter K. *Stockley's Drug Interactions.* 9th edn. London: Pharmaceutical Press: 2010
2. Bazire S. *Psychotropic Drug Directory 2012.* Stratford-upon-Avon; Lloyd-Reinhold Communications LLP: 2012
3. Clozaril specific product characteristics (SPC). Novartis. www.medicines.org.uk (accessed 15 November 2011)
4. Taylor D, Paton C, Kapur S. *The Maudsley Prescribing guidelines.* 10th edn: London: informa healthcare: 2010
5. Taylor D (1997) Pharmacokinetic interactions involving clozapine. *Br J Psychiatry* **171:** 109–12
6. Sandson N, Cozza K, Armstrong S, Eckermann G, Fischer B, Phillips B. Med-Psych Drug interaction update. Clozapine case series. *Psychosomatics* 2007; **48:** 170–5
7. Phillips KA, Veenstra DL, Oren E, Lee JK, Sadee W. Potential role of pharmacogeomics in reducing adverse drug reactions: a systematic review. *J Am Med Assoc* 2001; **286:** 2270–9
8. De Leon J, Armstrong S, Cozza K. Clinical guidelines for psychiatrists for the use of pharmacogenetic testing for CYP450 2D6 and CYP450 2C19. *Psychosomatics* 2006; **47:** 75–85
9. De Leon J. Respiratory infections rather than antibiotics may increase clozapine levels: A critical review of the literature. *J Clin Psychiatry* 2004; **65:** 1144–5
10. Lowe E, Ackman M. Impact of tobacco smoking cessation on stable clozapine or olanzapine treatment. *Ann Pharmacother* 2010; **44:** 727–32
11. Jann M, Grimsley S, Gray E, Chang Wen-Ho. Pharmacokinetics and pharmacodynamics of clozapine. *Clin Pharmacokinet* 1993; **24:** 161–76
12. Schaber G, Stevens I, Gaertner H, Dietz K, Breyer-Pfaff U. Pharmacokinetics of clozapine and its metabolites in psychiatric patients: plasma protein binding and renal clearance. *Br J Pharmacol* 1998; **46:** 453–9

9. Cancer chemotherapy

Approximately one in three people will develop cancer at some point during their lifetime[1]. Those with schizophrenia have a similar risk overall, with lung and breast cancer (in women) being found more frequently than the general population and skin and prostate cancer less frequently[2]. Given this common disease and the widespread use of clozapine, it is likely that many patients on clozapine will develop cancer at some point during treatment. This poses a clinical conundrum if the treatment of choice for the cancer is chemotherapy. Clozapine is formally contraindicated with other drugs which cause neutropenia, however discontinuing clozapine before chemotherapy may destabilise a patient who has taken many months or years to find symptom control. In the authors' clinical experience, those who become mentally unwell may retract consent for either chemotherapy or the re-introduction of clozapine, are less likely to comply with complex cancer treatments and may no longer attend follow-up appointments.

There are a number of case reports supporting continuing clozapine during chemotherapy (*Table 9.1*). From the limited case reports it does not appear that there is a synergistic effect or worsening of haematological outcome with the combination of clozapine and chemotherapy.

Recommendations

- Ideally, clozapine should be discontinued before the start of chemotherapy.
- This comes with a considerable risk of destabilising a patient who may then refuse consent for chemotherapy or a re-challenge with clozapine.
- The risks and benefits of stopping clozapine should be fully discussed with the patient, carer, mental health team, oncology service, clozapine monitoring service and pharmacy teams.
- Consider delaying chemotherapy until after the first three months of clozapine treatment.
- If continuing clozapine is in the best interest of the patient, rescue therapy such as granulocyte colony stimulating factor (GCSF) and increased haematological monitoring should be considered.
- Educate the patient and carers to report immediately any signs or symptoms of infection.

Table 9.1: Case reports of continuing clozapine during chemotherapy

Author	Diagnosis	Clozapine dose, mg/day	Clozapine duration	Lowest white blood cell count	Chemotherapy	Comments
Avnon et al, 1993[3]	Carcinoma of the uteral endometrium	125mg	2 years	Reported as suffered leucopenia	Not reported	
Frieri el at, 2008[4]	Non-Hodgkin lymphoma	300mg	6 years	2006, 630mm[3]	2002, 9 then 6 cycles of chlorambucil 2006, four cycles of fludarabine and mitoxantrone followed by cyclophosamide, vincristine and prednisolone	Clozapine was initially stopped in 2002 but then restarted.
Goulet et al, 2008[5]	Small cell lung cancer with hepatic metastases	300mg	10 years	3.0x109/L	6 cycles of cisplatin and etoposide	
Hundertmark et al, 2001[6]	Lymphoma	Not reported	Not reported	Reported as significant neutropenia	Not reported	Clozapine was reintroduced during chemotherapy
McKenna et al, 1994[7]	Small cell lung cancer	Not reported	Not reported	Not reported	Cisplatinum and etoposide	Only received 1 course of chemotherapy before withdrawing consent
Rosenberg et al, 2007[8]	Hodgkin's Lymphoma	600mg	10 years	0.1 cell/mm^3	Ablation chemotherapy and stem cell transplant	
Rosenstock, 2004[9]	Breast cancer	700mg	10 years	1.3x109/L	Four cycles of doxorubicin, cyclophosphamide and radiotherapy	Neutropenia continued for 6 months
Wesson et al, 1995[10]	Testicular teratoma with pulmonary metastases	Not reported	4 years	WBC 2.5x109/L	4 cycles of bleomycin, etoposide and cisplatin	Monitored white blood cell counts daily

Summary

- If possible, clozapine should be discontinued before chemotherapy.
- The risk of relapse and subsequent deterioration in mental health must be fully considered before discontinuation.
- If it is in the best interest of the patient to continue clozapine during chemotherapy, a collaborative approach between the oncology team, psychiatrist, patient, carer, pharmacy and clozapine service is strongly recommended.

References

1. Sasieni PD, Shelton J, Ormiston-Smith N, Thomson CS, Silcocks PB. What is the lifetime risk of developing cancer?: The effect of adjusting for multiple primaries. *Br J Cancer* 2011; **105:** 460–5
2. Catts VS, Catts SV, O'Toole BI, Frost ADJ. Cancer incidence in patients with schizophrenia and their first-degree relatives: a meta-analysis. *Acta Psychiatr Scand* 2008; **117:** 323–36
3. Avnon M, Stolerman I. Clozapine, Cancer and Schizophrenia. *Am J Psychiatry* 1993; **150:** 1562–3
4. Frieri T, Barzega G, Bada a, Villari V. Maintaining clozapine treatment during chemotherapy for non-Hodgkin's lymphoma. *Prog Neuropsychopharmacol Biol Psychiatry* 2008; **32:** 1611–12
5. Goulet K, Grignon S. Case report: clozapine given in the context of chemotherapy for lung cancer. *Psychooncology* 2008; **17:** 512–6
6. Hundertmark J, Campbell P. Reintroduction of clozapine after diagnosis of lymphoma. *Br J Psychiatry* 2001; **178:** 576
7. McKenna R, Bailey L, Haake J, Desai P, Prasad B. Clozapine and chemotherapy. *Hospital Community Psychiatry* 1994; **45:** 831
8. Rosenberg I, Mekinulov B, Cohen L, Galynker I. Restarting clozapine treatment during ablation chemotherapy and stem cell transplant for Hodgkin's Lymphoma. *Am J Psychiatry* 2007; **164:** 1438–9
9. Rosenstock J. Clozapine therapy during cancer treatment. *Am J Psychiatry* 2004; **161:** 175
10. Wesson M, Finnegan D, Clark P. Continuing clozapine despite neutropenia. *Br J Psychiatry* 1996; **168:** 217–20

10. Prescribing in complex patient groups

10.1: Pregnancy

All pregnancies carry a degree of risk to both the mother and the foetus. The base rate for obstetric complications and congenital malformations in the general population lies between 2 and 4% (20–40 in 1000 pregnancies)[1]. When the woman has schizophrenia, there is evidence of poorer outcomes to the mother, fetus and infant[2]. Women with schizophrenia tend to receive less prenatal care, have poorer nutrition and have higher rates of alcohol misuse, drug misuse and smoking compared with women not diagnosed with schizophrenia[2]. This in part may explain the higher rates of stillbirths, malformations, infant deaths, intrauterine growth retardation, and preterm deliveries seen in infants born to mothers with schizophrenia[3].

Many women with schizophrenia experience parental difficulties, which may mean that they lose custody of their children, which may further affect the mental health of the mother and disrupt the development of the infant. In addition, an episode of psychosis during pregnancy is thought to double adverse pregnancy outcomes (including stillbirth and death)[4] and any period of extreme agitation or stress may increase the risk of malformations[5] and cause long-term cognitive and emotional problems in the child[6]. All these factors need careful thought even before the clinician considers the extra risks incurred when using antipsychotics such as clozapine during pregnancy.

Does clozapine affect fertility?

Clozapine does not appear to directly affect fertility and, in fact, may increase it if the woman is switching to clozapine from a high potency antipsychotic which has previously caused hyperprolactinaemia. Clozapine can however, have indirect effects such as increased weight and hyperinsulinaemia, which may contribute to polycystic ovary syndrome and irregular menstruation[7].

Clozapine use during pregnancy

No antipsychotic can be considered completely safe in pregnancy because robust randomised studies investigating birth outcomes would be unethical. In general, first generation antipsychotics such as chlorpromazine, trifluoperazine and haloperidol have the most data or experience to support their safe use during pregnancy[8, 9, 10]. However, these would not be appropriate or effective for the majority of clozapine users.

Clozapine has not been shown to be a teratogen in either human[8, 9, 11] or animal studies[10], but data relating to pregnancy outcomes are limited to case reports or small prospective studies (*Table 10.1.1*). The rate of spontaneous abortions in women exposed to clozapine does not appear to be higher than that seen in the general population[12].

Table 10.1.1: Case reports and case series of clozapine exposure during pregnancy

	Number of cases reported (age of mother)	Dose of clozapine	Duration of clozapine treatment	Concurrent factors	Outcomes	Comment
Duran et al, 2008[14]	3 exposures, 2 mothers (-)	Both 200mg/day	Throughout pregnancy	Both mothers had a BMI within the normal rage	Normal birth, full term, no complications	–
Reis et al, 2008[15]	18 (-)	*	First trimester exposure only	Other drugs prescribed concurrently	One case of ectopic anus reported in the clozapine cohort. No gestational diabetes reported in the clozapine group	Data taken from the Swedish Medical Birth register, looked at all antipsychotics used in pregnancy
Mendhekar, 2007[16]	1 (30)	100mg/day	Throughout pregnancy	Good nutrition/engagement by mother	Normal pregnancy, no perinatal complications	Normal development by baby except delayed speech which continued up to 5 years of age
Klys et al, 2007[17]	1 (27)	*	Discontinued by the mental health team in the first trimester	Deliberate overdose with the intention of committing suicide at 9 months pregnant (ingested 100-200 x 100mg tablets)	Neonate died on delivery 25 hours after the overdose. Mother survived	The authors concluded it was safer to continue clozapine during pregnancy than discontinue
Sethi, 2006[18]	1 (20)	250mg / day	Throughout pregnancy		No complications	No develop-mental delay in child reported to 2 years

Table 10.1.1: Case reports and case series of clozapine exposure during pregnancy *continued*

	Number of cases reported (age of mother)	Dose of clozapine	Duration of clozapine treatment	Concurrent factors	Outcomes	Comment
Dickson et al, 1998[24]	1 (28)	Reduced during pregnancy from 450mg to 150mg/day	Throughout pregnancy	Clozapine-induced diabetes developed before pregnancy. Shoulder dystocia reported during delivery	No other complication reported	Fertility increase reported after starting clozapine
Nguyen et al, 2003[22]	2 exposures same mother (33 and 37)	350mg/day	Throughout pregnancy		Gestational diabetes developed during the first pregnancy (treated with insulin)	No developmental delay in children up to 5 years
McKenna et al, 2005[19]	6 (-)	*	First trimester and throughout pregnancy	Other drugs prescribed concurrently	No malformation seen in the clozapine group. A lower birth weight was seen in the atypical antipsychotic exposed group. Otherwise no significant difference in pregnancy outcomes versus the control group	Part of a larger prospective study into atypical antipsychotics during pregnancy
Gupta et al, 2004[20]	2 (25, -) exposures, same mother	100–200mg/day	Throughout pregnancy	Pregnancy induced hypertension at 38th week during the first birth, week 30 during second	Normal postnatal period	Normal development reported to 20 months (first birth), and 6 months (second birth)

Table 10.1.1: Case reports and case series of clozapine exposure during pregnancy *continued*

	Number of cases reported (age of mother)	Dose of clozapine	Duration of clozapine treatment	Concurrent factors	Outcomes	Comment
Karakula et al, 2004[21]	1 (29)	200mg/day	Throughout pregnancy	Early uterine contractions and delivered in the 28th week of pregnancy. Alcohol misuse in father	Multiple complications in infant: floppy infant syndrome, convulsions, CNS under observation, missing left testicle	Delayed development at 7 months. Authors suggest structural changes in the infant's testicles may indicate a possible teratogenic effect of clozapine
Yogev et al, 2002[23]	1 (31)	*	Throughout pregnancy	Uterine contractions at 34 weeks which resolved, delivery at 37 weeks	A temporary decreased foetal heart rate variability was noted. Otherwise pregnancy and delivery normal	The authors suggest that clozapine may have temporary affected the foetal CNS
Stoner et al, 1997[25]	2 (30, 32)	Case 1: 300mg/day Case 2: 600–625mg/day	Periods of non-compliance reported in both cases which contributed to psychotic symptoms worsening	Both cases report lithium exposure during the first trimester	Case 1: infant experienced a seizure 8 days after birth due to gastroenteritis and mild gastroesopageal reflux disease Case 2: postpartum low grade fever in infant	Case 1: no developmental problems up to 2 years
Di Michele et al, 1996[26]	1 (37)	200–300mg/day	Throughout pregnancy	Also on lorazepam 2.5mg 3–5 times a day throughout pregnancy	Infant had benign tachypnoea and mild floppy infant syndrome on delivery. Resolved 5 days later	Uneventful pregnancy

Table 10.1.1: Case reports and case series of clozapine exposure during pregnancy *continued*

	Number of cases reported (age of mother)	Dose of clozapine	Duration of clozapine treatment	Concurrent factors	Outcomes	Comment
Walderman et al 1993[27]	1 (30)	*	Throughout pregnancy	Shoulder dystocia reported during delivery	Gestational diabetes developed in second trimester, otherwise uneventful	No exacerbation of psychosis noted during pregnancy, labour or delivery. The authors cited 14 other women who had taken clozapine during gestation with no apparent adverse effects to mother or foetus
Barnas et al, 1994[28]	1 (31)	50–100mg/day	Throughout pregnancy	Clozapine plasma levels were taken monthly during pregnancy	Uneventful pregnancy except weight gain (25kg)	No psychomotor abnormalities reported at 6 months

* – not reported

The UK authorities however, suggest that clozapine should not be routinely prescribed in pregnancy (because of the theoretical risk of agranulocytosis in the foetus) and that the clinician should consider switching to another drug with careful monitoring[1]. Unfortunately, for the majority of women on clozapine, switching to another antipsychotic will not provide adequate efficacy and place them at a high risk of relapse. The FDA in the US classifies clozapine as category B[13], which means that there is no evidence of an increased risk of foetal abnormalities in humans.

Of the 42 case reports of clozapine exposure during pregnancy there are two reports of congenital abnormalities (one structural change in the testicles[25] and one ectopic anus[26]). In all the other cases clozapine appeared to present no increased risk of malformations. A summary of other complications reported during pregnancy which were possibly related to clozapine exposure can be seen in *Table 10.1.2*.

Clozapine plasma levels during pregnancy

There are no published studies investigating changes in clozapine or norclozapine levels during pregnancy. Barnas et al conducted monthly clozapine plasma levels in their patient during pregnancy and reported clozapine levels between 38 and 55ng/ml while prescribed 100mg/day, and 14.1 and 15.4ng/ml on 50mg/day[16]. Theoretically, one may expect a reduction in clozapine levels due to an increased plasma volume and increased CYP2D6 and 3A4 metabolism during pregnancy, but this may be counterbalanced by an increase in protein binding and a reduction in CYP1A2 enzymatic activity[29]. Until more extensive studies are available, clozapine levels should be monitored monthly throughout pregnancy and repeated a week after delivery.

Table 10.1.2: A summary of the complications reported during pregnancy and immediately after delivery following clozapine exposure

No of cases	Complication
1	Pregnancy-induced hypertension[20]
2	Gestational diabetes[22,27]
2	Shoulder dystocia[24,27]
1	A seizure eight days after birth (gastroenteritis may have contributed)[25]
1	A low grade fever in the infant[25]
1	Benign tachypnoea in the infant[26]
2	Floppy infant syndrome[21,26] (in one case a high dose of regular lorazepam may have contributed)
1	Decreased foetal heart rate variability[23]

Table 10.1.3 (overleaf) provides a summary of other factors to consider when using clozapine during pregnancy.

Overall, the majority of case reports describe a largely uneventful pregnancy with normal development of the child on follow-up (up to five years). Interpreting case reports however, is fraught with difficulty and must be approached with caution. They are often biased towards adverse outcomes and may have incomplete details. While the literature is encouraging, clozapine should be used with caution in pregnancy.

Summary

- Clozapine is not considered a human teratogen but the data reporting pregnancy outcomes and later child development are limited to case reports or small prospective studies.
- Discontinuing clozapine during or before pregnancy entails a considerable risk of relapse, which may incur a greater risk to the mother and child than the risk of continued effective use during pregnancy.
- In all individuals, risk-benefit analysis should be conducted.
- Due to the unpredictable pharmacokinetics of clozapine during pregnancy, monitor plasma levels monthly then repeat a week after the birth.

- Maintain clozapine on the lowest effective dose during pregnancy and avoid concurrent medication, where possible.
- Always seek expert advice and gather the latest evidence, ideally before the woman becomes pregnant.
- Engage both partners in a frank, open discussion about the risks of clozapine in pregnancy and fully document such discussions.

Table 10.1.3. General principles of prescribing clozapine in pregnancy (adapted with permission from the *Maudsley Guidelines* 11th edition)[8]

In all women of child-bearing potential on clozapine: ▸ Always discuss the possibilities of pregnancy (those with schizophrenia have a higher risk of unplanned pregnancies than the general population)[1] and discuss adequate contraception methods ▸ If switching from a high potency antipsychotic to clozapine, consider if fertility will now increase
If a woman taking clozapine is considering becoming pregnant: ▸ Consider completing a medication review to investigate if any other antipsychotic with more extensive evidence in pregnancy has been successfully trialled ▸ Refer to specialist perinatal services to ensure that you have the latest advice on clozapine in pregnancy ▸ If smoking, encourage smoking cessation and consider appropriate nicotine replacement therapy (remember smoking cessation can dramatically increase clozapine levels ▸ Monitor closely for worsening diabetes or emerging gestational diabetes (consider monthly blood glucose levels) ▸ Ensure adequate folate supplementation and encourage attendance at antenatal appointments and screening
If a woman taking clozapine discovers that she is pregnant (also see advice above): ▸ Abrupt discontinuation of clozapine is unwise because of the increased risk of relapse which is likely to be more harmful than continued effective treatment ▸ Switching to another antipsychotic exposes the foetus to another drug and may not be fully effective. Remaining on clozapine may be in the best interests of both the mother and infant
In all pregnant women who are taking clozapine: ▸ Ensure the parents and partners are involved (where possible) in all decisions and supply them with appropriate written advice ▸ Try to avoid all drugs during the first trimester (when major organs are being formed), unless the benefit outweighs the risk. This is unlikely to be possible in the majority of clozapine users ▸ Use the lowest effective clozapine dose ▸ Prescribe as few drugs as possible both simultaneously and in sequence with clozapine ▸ Monitor clozapine plasma levels monthly and adjust the dose accordingly. Note blood volume and hepatic enzyme activity change markedly during pregnancy ▸ Monitor closely for other side-effects of clozapine which may be exacerbated in pregnancy (e.g. weight gain, constipation, sedation, orthostatic hypotension) ▸ Inform the obstetric team of clozapine use and possible complications to the mother (e.g. diabetes) and neonate (e.g. floppy infant syndrome) ▸ Fully document all decisions and advice given

References

1. National Institute for Health and Clinical Excellence. *Antenatal and Postnatal Mental Health, Clinical Guideline 45*. Available at: http://www.nice.org.uk . 2007 (accessed August 2012)
2. Yaeger D, Smith H, Altshuler L. Atypical antipsychotics in the treatment of schizophrenia during pregnancy and the postpartum. *Am J Psychiatry* 2006; **163:** 2064–70
3. Howard L. Fertility and pregnancy in women with psychotic disorders. *Eur J Obst Gynecol Reprod Biol* 2006; **178:** 427–32
4. Nilsson E, Lichtenstein P, Cnattingius S, Murray RM, Hultman CM. Women with schizophrenia: pregnancy outcome and infant death among their offspring. *Schizophr Res* 2002; **58:** 221–9
5. Hansen D, Lou HC, Olsen J. Serious life events and congenital malformations: a national study with complete follow up. *Lancet* 2000; **356:** 875–80
6. Talge N, Neal C, Glover V. Antenatal maternal stress and long-term effects on child neurodevelopment: how and why? *J Child Psychol Psychiatry* 2007; **48:** 245–61
7. Ernst CL, Goldberg J. The reproductive safety profile of mood stabilizers, atypical antipsychotics, and broad spectrum psychotropics. *J Clin Psychiatry* 2002; **63 Suppl 4:** 42–55
8. Taylor D, Paton C, Kapur S. *The Maudsley Prescribing guidelines.* 11th edn: Oxford: Wiley-Blackwell: 2012
9. Bazire S. *Psychotropic Drug Directory 2012*. Stratford-upon-Avon: Lloyd-Reinhold Communications: 2012
10. Gentile S. Antipsychotic therapy during early and late pregnancy. A systematic review. *Schizophr Bull* 2010; **36:** 518–44
11. Briggs G, Freeman R, Yaffe S. *Drugs in Pregnancy and Lactation*. 9th revised edn: Philadelphia: Lippincott Williams and Wilkins: 2011
12. Gentile S. Clinical utilization of atypical antipsychotics in pregnancy and lactation. *Ann Pharmacother* 2004; **38:** 1265–71
13. Clozaril prescribing information. Available at: www.fda.gov (accessed14 August 2012)
14. Duran A, Ugur M, Turan S, Emul M. Clozapine use in two women with schizophrenia during pregnancy. *J Psychopharmacol* 2008; **22:** 111–13
15. Reis M, Källén B. Maternal use of antipsychotics in early pregnancy and delivery outcome. *J Clin Psychopharmacol* 2008; **28:** 279–88
16. Mendhekar D. Possible delayed speech acquisition with clozapine therapy during pregnancy and lactation. *J Neuropsychiatry Clin Neurosci* 2007; **19:** 196–7
17. Klys M, Rojek S, Rzepecka-Wozniak E. Neonatal death following clozapine self-poisoning in late pregnancy. *Forensic Sci Int* 2007; **171:** e5–e10.
18. Sethi S. Clozapine in pregnancy. Indian Journal of Psychiatry 2006: 48; 196-197
19. McKenna K, Koren G, Tetelbaum M, Wilton L, Shakir S, Diav-Citrin O, et al. Pregnancy outcome of women using atypical antipsychotic drugs: a prospective comparative study. *J Clin Psychiatry* 2005; **66:** 444–9
20. Gupta N, Grover S. Safety of clozapine in 2 successive pregnancies. *Can J Psychiatry* 2004; **49:** 863
21. Karakula H, Szajer K, Spila B, Grzywa A, Chuchra M. Clozapine and pregnancy: A case history. *Pharmacopsychiatry* 2004; **37:** 303–4
22. Nguyen H, Lalonde P. Clozapine in pregnancy. *L'Encephale* 2003; **29:** 119–24
23. Yogev Y, Ben-Haroush A, Kaplan B. Maternal clozapine treatment and decreased fetal heart rate

variability. *Int J Gynaecol Obstet* 2002; **79:** 259–60

24. Dickson R, Hogg L. Pregnancy of a patient treated with clozapine. *Psychiatr Serv* 1998; **49:** 1081–3.
25. Stoner S, Sommi R, Marken P, Anya I, Vaughn J. Clozapine use in two full-term pregnancies. *J Clin Psychiatry* 1997; **58:** 364–5
26. Di Michele V, Ramenghi L, Sabatino G. Clozapine and lorazepam administration in pregnancy. *Eur Psychiatry* 1996; **11:** 214
27. Barnas C, Bergant A, Hummer M, Saria A, Wolfgang Fleischhacker W. Clozapine concentrations in maternal and fetal plasma, amniotic fluid, and breast milk. *Am J Psychiatry* 1994; **6:** 945
28. Walderman M, Safferman A. Pregnancy and clozapine. *Am J Psychiatry* 1993; **150:** 168–9
29. Anderson G. Pregnancy induced changes in pharmacokinetics: A mechanistic based approach. *Clin Pharmacokinet* 2005; **44:** 989–1008

10.2: Breastfeeding

The vast benefits of breastfeeding to both mother and child are well documented and most authorities recommend exclusive breastfeeding for at least the first six months of life[1]. Although more than half of breastfeeding women take some type of medication while feeding[2], information on the use of almost any medication during breastfeeding is scarce, with most data coming from case reports or small case series[3]. There are few data supporting use of antipsychotics during breastfeeding[3]. For clozapine, there are only two, fully available published case reports.

In the first, Barnas et al in 1994 reported on a 31-year-old who received 50mg–100mg of clozapine throughout pregnancy. The pregnancy was largely uneventful and although the woman did not breastfeed, clozapine levels were taken in the mother, foetus and breast milk on day one and seven days after delivery. The day after delivery the clozapine plasma level in the mother was 14.7ng/ml and in the first portion of breast milk was 63.5ng/ml (at a clozapine dose of 50mg per day). At one week after delivery, the mother's plasma level was 41.4ng/ml and the breast milk concentration was 115.6ng/ml (at a clozapine dose of 100mg per day). This represents a milk to plasma ratio (M/P) of 2.8 and suggests that the infant would receive about 173mcgs/kg of clozapine daily, or 1% of the maternal weight-related dose[5].

A concentration of drug in the milk which exceeds that found in the plasma (M/P >1) suggests significant exposure to the infant[6]. Conversely, an infant plasma concentration of 10% or less of the therapeutic level in the mother is often considered acceptable[6]. As clozapine has a relatively low molecular weight (C18H19ClN4 = 326.87) and high lipid solubility, extensive passage into breast milk would be expected[6].

In the second report, the author presented a 30-year-old who took 100mg of clozapine throughout pregnancy and while breastfeeding[8]. The pregnancy was uneventful and the mother breastfed the baby until one-year-old. The infant had normal development except for delayed speech. At three years the infant spoke only 12–15 words and exhibited stuttering. Intervention by a speech and language therapist did not appear to elicit much response. By the age of five years however, the speech impairment had resolved. The author reported no other contributing factors to the speech impairment, although clozapine exposure during pregnancy may have been important.

There are further less-detailed case studies suggesting that babies exposed to clozapine while being breastfed have experienced sedation[5], agranulocytosis[9], cardiovascular instability[10], decreased suckling reflex, irritability and seizures[11]. However, details on these reports have not been published in full. There are also two case reports of there being no adverse effects in infants exposed to clozapine during breastfeeding[11]. Again, full details of these cases are not available.

Table 10.2.1 presents a summary of the case reports investigating the effects of clozapine while breastfeeding. Caution is advocated when interpreting case reports: they often only report adverse outcomes, may be limited in detail, and effects cannot definitely be separated from the maternal exposure of the drug.

Table 10.2.1: Summary of the case reports investigating the effects of clozapine while breastfeeding

Milk to plasma ratio of clozapine	Infant dose vs. mother dose	Adverse effects reported in infants exposed to clozapine during breastfeeding
2.84 (above 1 is considered significant exposure)	1%[4] (below 10% is often considered acceptable)	▸ Delayed speech acquisition[7] ▸ Sedation[5] ▸ Agranulocytosis[9] ▸ Cardiovascular instability[10] ▸ Decreased sucking reflex[11] ▸ Irritability[11] ▸ Seizures[11]

Table 10.2.2: General points to consider when continuing medication during breastfeeding[11, 14]

- Each case must be assessed individually, weighing the benefits of breastfeeding to the mother and child against the risk of drug exposure to the infant
- The infant should be closely monitored for any drug-related adverse effects and delays in development
- Preterm babies represent a higher risk than full-term babies because of underdeveloped organs
- Drugs are mainly transferred into breast-milk by passive diffusion. Small molecules which are very lipid soluble (such as clozapine) diffuse rapidly
- Hind-milk has a higher fat content than fore-milk, so can further concentrate lipid soluble drugs
- The ability to metabolise drugs in the infant is limited in the first few weeks of life (because of an underdeveloped hepatic function)
- Use the lowest effective dose of medication and avoid polypharmacy where possible

UK authorities recommend that clozapine should not be routinely prescribed for women who are breastfeeding (because it reaches high levels in breast milk and there is a risk of agranulocytosis in the infant)[12]. The American Academy of Pediatrics classifies clozapine as a drug whose effect on the nursing infant is unknown but may be of concern[13]. Unfortunately, those on clozapine are unlikely to be successfully transferred to another antipsychotic or be suitable for a drug free period. So, the question in practice is usually should the mother breastfeed while continuing clozapine? Until more data become available, breastfeeding should be avoided while being prescribed clozapine, although this decision may be unacceptable to some women. Decisions should be made on a case-by-case basis, involving both parents in discussions where possible. Given the low concentrations of clozapine in milk (at least low enough to limit infant exposure to minute levels), adverse effects might be considered unlikely. However, neutropenia is not dose-dependent and so the risk of blood dyscrasia in the infant is not reduced. *Table 10.2.2* outlines general points to consider when continuing medication while breastfeeding.

Summary

- There are only a handful of case reports documenting the outcome to babies exposed to clozapine during breastfeeding.
- Clozapine is significantly excreted into breast milk, at a milk to plasma ratio of 2.8. This may equate to the infant receiving approximately 1% of the mother's dose.
- Adverse events reported in the infant following exposure to clozapine in breast milk are delayed speech acquisition, sedation, agranulocytosis, cardiovascular instability, decreased suckling reflex, irritability and seizures.
- Until more data become available, breastfeeding should be avoided while being prescribed clozapine.
- Clozapine should not be stopped to allow breastfeeding.

Free on-line resource

Drugs and lactation database (LactMed). From the United States National Library of Medicine. Available at: http://toxnet.nlm.nih.gov/

References

1. WHO/UNICEF. Global strategy for infant and young child feeding. Geneva, Switzerland: World Health Organization; 2003. Available at: www.who.int. (accessed 16 August 2012)
2. Sultz E, Stokes J, Shaffer M, Paul I, Berlin C. Extent of medication use in breastfeeding women. *Breastfeeding Med* 2007; **2:** 145–51
3. Fortinguerra F, Clavenna A, Bonati M. Psychotropic drug use during breastfeeding : A review of the evidence. *Pediatrics* 2009; **124:** e547–e556
4. Barnas C, Bergant A, Hummer M, Saria A, Wolfgang Fleischhacker W. Clozapine concentrations in maternal and fetal plasma, amniotic fluid, and breast milk. *Am J Psychiatry* 1994; **6:** 945
5. Schaefer C, Peters P, Miller R. *Drugs during Pregnancy and Lactation: Treatment options and risk assessment.* 2nd edn: London: Academic Press Inc: 2007
6. Menon S. Psychotropic medication during pregnancy and lactation. *Arch Gynecol Obstet* 2008; **277:** 1–13
7. Royal Pharmaceutical Society, Sweetman S. *Martindale: the complete drug reference.* 37th edn. London: Pharmaceutical Press: 2011
8. Mendhekar D. Possible delayed speech acquisition with clozapine therapy during pregnancy and lactation. *J Neuropsychiatry Clin Neurosci* 2007; **19:** 196–7
9. Gentile S. Clinical utilization of atypical antipsychotics in pregnancy and lactation. *Ann Pharmacother*

2004; **38:** 1265–71

10. Iqbal M, Rahman A, Husain Z, Mahmud S, Ryan W, Feldman J. Clozapine: a clinical review of adverse effects and management. *Ann Clin Psychiatry* 2003; **15:** 33–48
11. Taylor D, Paton C, Kapur S. *The Maudsley Prescribing guidelines.* 11th edn: Oxford: Wiley-Blackwell: 2012
12. National Institute for Health and Clinical Excellence. *Antenatal and Postnatal Mental Health, Clinical Guideline* 45. Available at: http://www.nice.org.uk . 2007. (accessed August 2012)
13. Committee on Drugs, American Academy for Pediatrics. The transfer of drugs and other chemicals into human milk. *Pediatrics* 2001; **108:** 776–89
14. Yoshia K, Smith B, Kumar B. Psychotropic drugs in mothers' milk: a comprehensive review of assay methods, pharmacokinetics and safety of breast-feeding. *J Psychopharmacol* 1999; **13:** 64–80

10.3: Renal impairment

People with renal impairment have a reduced capacity to excrete drugs and their metabolites, and so need to be treated with considerable caution. Altered pharmacokinetics in renal impairment can result in accumulation of the drug, which may cause adverse effects and serious toxicity. Drugs which are extensively excreted by the kidneys, nephrotoxic, long-acting, or cause urinary retention are particularly problematic and should be avoided where possible. Despite being largely hepatically deactivated, clozapine has many adverse reactions which can contribute to or worsen renal impairment. Monitoring renal function is therefore advised before initiating clozapine and at least annually thereafter.

Measuring renal function

In clinical practice, renal function is measured by using serum creatinine and a prediction formula to give an estimation of creatinine clearance. The two most commonly used formulae are the Cockcroft and Gault equation and the 4-variable Modification of Diet in Renal Disease (MDRD) formula (*Figure 10.3.1*).

Figure 10.3.1: The Cockroft and Gault equation and the 4-v MDRD[1, 2]

The Cockroft and Gault equation

Estimated creatinine clearance

$$\text{CrCl (ml/min)} = \frac{(140\text{-age}) \times \text{weight} \times 1.2}{\text{serum creatinine}} \times 0.85 \text{ if femalc}$$

Age is expressed in years, serum creatinine in µmol/L and weight in kg

4-variable MDRD (adjusted for a body surface area of $1.73m^3$)

$186.3\text{x (Serum creatinine/88.4)}^{-1.154} \times \text{age}^{-0.203} \times (0.742 \text{ if female}) \times (1.21 \text{ if black})$

Age is expressed in years and serum creatinine in µmol/L

Most laboratories routinely report the estimated glomerular filtration rates (eGFR) using the 4-variable MDRD. Estimated GFR is less accurate in certain patient groups, such as those with a muscle wasting disorder, those with a rapidly changing renal function, acute renal failure, pregnancy or those who have severe malnutrition[1]. In these patient groups, specialist advice should be sought. More formal and accurate ways of measuring creatinine clearance such as urine collection over 24 hours, radioisotopic or radiocontrast agents are occasionally utilised by specialists[1].

The clinical relevance of eGFR and the stages of chronic renal disease can be seen in *Table 10.3.1*.

Table 10.3.1: The stages of chronic kidney disease[1,2,3]

Estimated glomerular filtration rate (eGFR) ml/min/1.73m²	Clinical significance/recommendations	Stage of chronic kidney disease
≥ 90	Normal function or stage 1 with other evidence of chronic kidney disease*	1
60–89	Slight decrease in GFR (mild impairment) consider normal unless other evidence of kidney disease*	2
45–59	Moderate impairment, evaluate and treat complications. Consider referral to specialists	3A
30–44		3B
15–29	Severe impairment, urgent referral to specialists, consider renal replacement	4
<15 (or receiving dialysis)	Established renal failure	5

* other evidence of chronic renal damage includes persistent proteinuria or haematuria or both, microalbuminuria in patients with diabetes or structural kidney disease

Clozapine in renal impairment

Clozapine is almost completely metabolised before excretion. Thus, only trace amounts of unchanged clozapine (around 0.12%)[4] are excreted in the urine. Approximately 50% of the metabolised drug (mainly as clozapine-N-oxide, whose activity is not known)[4] is excreted in the urine[5]. Based on these pharmacokinetic properties, clozapine (as the parent molecule) would not be expected to accumulate extensively in those with renal impairment. *Table 10.3.2* presents suggestions (from renal experts) on how to dose clozapine in renal impairment. It is important to note that clozapine is contraindicated in severe renal impairment by the manufacturer, although this is likely to be because of a lack of supporting evidence. There is only one case report investigating clozapine and norclozapine levels before and after haemodialysis[6]. In this study neither clozapine nor norclozapine levels (or ratios) changed during haemodialysis[6]. This single report suggests clozapine may not be actively dialysed.

Clozapine can cause or worsen diabetes (*Chapter 5.2*), which increases the risk of renal impairment. Other clozapine-related adverse reactions which may worsen symptoms of renal impairment include nocturnal enuresis, urinary retention, sedation and hypotension.

Interstitial nephritis

Clozapine has been reported to cause acute interstitial nephritis (AIN), although rarely (*Table 10.3.3* shows the case reports[9–14]). Although rare, AIN is an important cause of acute renal failure and is most often caused by medication[15]. Clozapine-induced AIN, as with other medication, appears to occur early on in treatment (usually within the first three weeks) and is independent of dose[16]. Withdrawing clozapine immediately and referring to specialists for advice is essential in suspected AIN to avoid chronic renal impairment and further complications. As AIN is thought to be a cell-mediated immune response[16], re-challenging with clozapine following AIN is likely to produce a similar or potentially worse reactions and thus should be not be undertaken.

Table 10.3.2: Suggested clozapine dosing in renal impairment[7]

	Clozapine dosing
eGFR ≥11	Use with caution, but dose as if normal renal function
eGFR <10 (or dialysis)	Use with caution. Start with a low dose and titrate slowly (e.g. half to a quarter of normal dosing). Clozapine levels would be useful to guide dosing[8]
Continuous ambulatory peritoneal dialysis (CAPD)/haemodialysis	Unlikely to be dialysed, dose as for eGFR <10mL/min
Intermittent haemodiafiltration	Unknown dialysability, dose as in GFR<10 mL/min
Continuous arteriovenous/veno-venous haemodialysis	Unknown dialysability, dose as in eGFR <10 mL/min

Table 10.3.3: Case reports of clozapine-induced interstitial nephritis

Author	Age/sex	Daily dose of clozapine	Duration of clozapine treatment	Symptoms/comments
Hunter et al, 2009[9]	57, female	25mg	4 days	Tachycardia, pyrexia, protein and RBCs in the urine. Clozapine was stopped on day 4. On day 8 eGFR= 40ml/min/1.73m^2, which improved by day 9. During a previous trial on clozapine she also developed renal failure
Siddiqui et al, 2008[10]	26, male	125mg	14 days	Fever, hypertension, eosinophilia. The serum creatinine was 133μmol/L. He was treated with IV hydration and IV steroids. He also developed cardiomyopathy
Au et al, 2004[11]	33, male	100mg	14 days	Nausea, vomiting, sore throat, diarrhoea, fever and a positive urinalysis (which included WBCs, protein and haemoglobin). His creatinine level was 857μmol/L and the diagnosis of acute renal failure was made. Treatment included IV hydration and antibiotics. Over one week his renal function improved

Table 10.3.3: Case reports of clozapine-induced interstitial nephritis *continued*

Author	Age/ sex	Daily dose of clozapine	Duration of clozapine treatment	Symptoms/comments
Southall et al, 2000[12]	24, female	300mg	12 days	Tachycardia, pyrexia, nausea and vomiting, raised urine protein and eosinophilia. Symptoms settled within 24 hours of stopping clozapine. Renal function tests remained normal throughout the episode
Fraser et al, 2000[13]	49, male	Not reported	35 days	Acute confusion and pyrexia. Renal impairment returned on re-exposure to clozapine. Treatment included peritoneal dialysis followed by haemodialysis and IV methylphenidate. Renal biopsy confirmed interstitial nephritis
Elias et al, 1999[14]	38, female	250mg	11 days	The patient had no history of pre-existing renal disease but was concurrently prescribed lithium 750mg daily. Symptoms included anorexia, lethargy, vomiting and reduced urine output. Her urea was 32.9mmol/l and creatinine 1200μmol/L on admission to hospital. Following intermittent haemodialysis her renal function returned to normal after 15 days

Summary

- Clozapine is almost completely metabolised before excretion. Only trace amounts of unchanged clozapine is excreted in the urine.
- Clozapine would not be expected to accumulate extensively in those with renal impairment, but (possibly because there is no supporting literature) the manufacturer contraindicates clozapine in severe renal impairment.
- It would seem prudent to titrate clozapine slowly and use lower initial doses in those with renal impairment.
- Many adverse reactions associated with clozapine can contribute to or worsen renal impairment (e.g. diabetes, urinary retention and hypotension).
- There are case reports of clozapine causing interstitial nephritis. This constitutes a medical emergency where clozapine must be immediately stopped and expert advice sought. Re-exposure to clozapine is contraindicated.
- Renal function should be measured before starting clozapine and then at least annually during treatment.

Web resource

The UK Renal Association provides expert guidance on interpreting results and treating chronic renal impairment. Available at: www.renal.org/egfr

References

1. Traynor J, Mactier R, Geddes C, Fox J. How to measure renal function in clinical practice. *Br Med J* 2006; **333:** 733–7
2. Stevens L, Coresh J, Greene T, Levey A. Assessing kidney function – measured and estimated glomerular filtration rate. *N Engl J Med* 2006; **354:** 2473–83
3. National Institute for Health and Clinical Excellence. *Chronic Kidney Disease, Clinical Guideline 73.* Available at: http://www.nice.org.uk . 2008 (accessed September 2012)
4. Schaber G, Stevens I, Gaertner H, Dietz K, Breyer-Pfaff U. Pharmacokinetics of clozapine and its metabolites in psychiatric patients: plasma protein binding and renal clearance. *Br J Clin Pharmacol* 1998; **46:** 453–9
5. Clozaril specific product characteristics (SPC). Novartis. Available at: www.medicines.org.uk (accessed September 2012)
6. Jacob A, Zahr N, Hulot JS, Boussouar S, Vilain J, Lafont-Rapnouil S, et al. Therapeutic drug monitoring of clozapine in a hemodialysed smoking patient with schizophrenia. *Ther Drug Monit* 2009; **31:** 281–2
7. Ashley C, Currie A. *The Renal Drug Handbook.* 3rd revised edn: Milton Keynes: Radcliffe Publishing Ltd: 2008
8. Taylor D, Paton C, Kapur S. *The Maudsley Prescribing guidelines.* 11th edn: Chichester: Wiley-Blackwell: 2012
9. Hunter R, Gaughan T, Queirazza F, McMillan D, Shankie S. Clozapine-induced interstitial nephritis — a rare but important complication: a case report. *J Med Case Reports* 2009; **3:** 8574
10. Siddiqui B, Asim S, Shamim A, Pillai N, Rajan S. Simultaneous allergic interstitial nephritis and cardiomyopathy in a patient on clozapine. *Nephrol Dial Transplant Plus* 2008; **1:** 55–6
11. Au A, Luthra V, Stern R. Clozapine-induced acute interstitial nephritis. *Am J Psychiatry* 2004; **161:** 1501
12. Southall K, Fernando S. A case of interstitial nephritis on clozapine. *Aust N Z J Psychiatry* 2000; **34:** 697–8
13. Fraser D, Jlbani M. An unexpected and seriour complication of treatment with the atypical antipsychotic drug clozapine. *Clin Nephrol* 2000; **54:** 78–80
14. Elias T, Bannister K, Clarkson A, Faull D, Faull R. Clozapine-induced interstitial nephritis. *Lancet* 1999; **354:** 1180–81
15. Kodner C, Kudrimoti A. Diagnosis and management of acute interstitial nephritis. *Am Fam Physician* 2003; **67:** 2527–34
16. Rossert J. Drug-induced acute interstitial nephritis. *Kidney Int* 2001; **60:** 804–17

10.4: Liver impairment

The liver plays a key role in the elimination of clozapine and its active and inactive metabolites. People with liver dysfunction are more sensitive to the adverse effects of clozapine because of reduced biotransformation, altered protein binding, reduced hepatic blood flow or altered biliary excretion[1]. Clozapine itself has been associated with elevated liver enzymes and acute liver disorders, such as toxic hepatitis and fulminant liver failure. In addition, some adverse effects of clozapine can complicate symptoms of both acute and chronic liver impairment.

Liver function should be a routine part of physical health monitoring, as clozapine is known to cause liver dysfunction and so dosage adjustments may be required.

Clozapine treatment in chronic liver impairment

Clozapine is subject to moderate first pass metabolism (absolute bioavailability of 50–60%)[2] and extensive protein binding (clozapine 95%, norclozapine 90% and clozapine-N-oxide 75%)[3]. Thus, in severe liver impairment, an accumulation of clozapine might be expected through a reduction in pre-systemic elimination and an increase in unbound clozapine. Clozapine is extensively metabolised by a variety of liver enzymes (*Figure 10.4.1*). These enzymes are compromised in liver disease, but the degree to which their function is reduced depends on the specific cytochrome, severity of liver disease and underlying fast or poor metabolising status of the person. Cytochrome P450 2C19 appears to be compromised in the early stages of hepatic dysfunction, but CYP1A2, 2D6 and 3A4 only in later, more severe stages of liver disease[1].

There is much inter-individual variation in the rate and extent of liver disease, so predicting exact dosing adjustments for clozapine is not possible. In general, those with cirrhosis are at particular risk as the number of functioning hepatocytes and thus

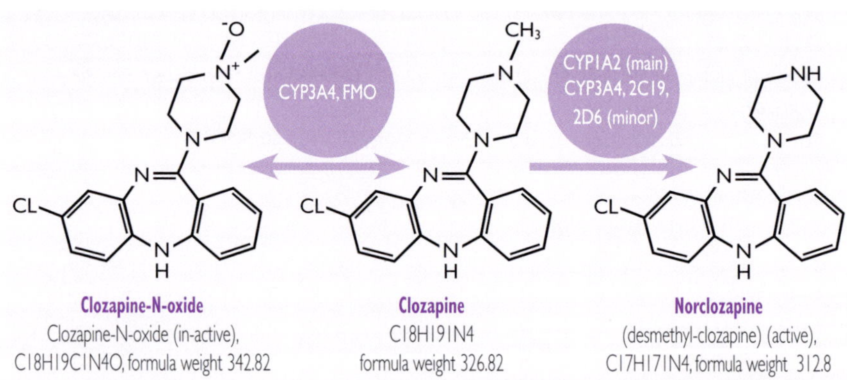

Figure 10.4.1: The main metabolic processes of clozapine[3, 5] (the ration of clozapine:norclozapine: clozapine-N-oxide is 1:1:2)

metabolising enzymes are reduced[1]. Other liver diseases without cirrhosis, such as chronic hepatitis, primary or secondary liver cancer and hepatosplenic schistomiasis are not usually associated with a clinically significant impaired metabolism, and are less likely to cause changes in drug kinetics[4].

The severity of liver disease is often rated according to the Child-Pugh classification (*Table 10.4.1*)[5], or the model for end-stage liver disease, MELD[1]. Unfortunately however, neither classification system is sensitive enough to be able to predict declining drug metabolising status, so they cannot be used as a guide to adjust doses. They do provide a rough guide to disease severity and may help highlight those who need closer monitoring and more cautious prescribing. Prothrombin time and plasma albumen are also used to indicate liver function (i.e if these parameters are normal then function is preserved). Of note is that in advanced liver disease, kidney function is also often compromised, which complicates further clozapine kinetics and may necessitate additional dosing adjustments and monitoring.

Table 10.4.1: The Child-Pugh classification[6]

Points	1	2	3
Encephalopathy	None	Minimal	Advanced (coma)
Ascities	Absent	Controlled	Refractory
Serum bilirubin (μmol/L)	<34	34–51	>51
Serum albumin (g/L)	>35	28–35	<28
Prothrombin (s)	<4	4–6	>6

Points are summed, and the total score is classified according to severity: 5–6 points = group A (mild); 7–9 points = B (moderate); 10–15 points = C (severe)

Clinicians should start with a low dose (e.g. 12.5mg daily) when initiating clozapine to those with liver disease and titrate slowly, using plasma levels to guide dosing. Any signs of intolerable adverse effects which may suggest accumulating clozapine or an excess of 'free' clozapine should be followed by a reduction or postponing of the titration. In particular, emerging constipation or sedation with clozapine should be immediately addressed to avoid precipitating hepatic encephalopathy[7]. Manufacturers of clozapine contraindicate its use in progressive liver disease, hepatic failure and active liver disease associated with nausea, anorexia or jaundice[2]. Liver function tests (LFTs) should be monitored before initiating clozapine and then repeated at least annually. Any signs or symptoms of liver impairment should prompt additional monitoring.

Clozapine as a cause of acute liver disorders

Clozapine (and most other antipsychotics[8, 9]) commonly increase concentrations of liver enzymes (the incidence with clozapine is around 30%[8, 10]). This increase usually occurs in the first six weeks of treatment, is transient in nature and is often asymptomatic[8]. Alanine aminotransferase (ALT) appears to be the enzyme most often and strongly affected[8] followed by aspartate aminotransferase (AST). In approximately 60% of cases, the enzyme elevation caused by clozapine spontaneously resolves without altering the dose or discontinuing treatment[8, 10]. Where spontaneous resolution occurs, this is usually achieved within 13 weeks of starting clozapine treatment[10]. Risk factors associated with this enzyme increase are unclear, but some authors suggest a higher dose and being male may be important factors[10]. The mechanism behind clozapine-associated idiosyncratic hepatic injury also remains unclear, but the latency period is consistent with a hypersensitivity reaction[11]. Clozapine may also contribute to obesity and type 2 diabetes, both of which are associated with a fatty liver and further increase the risk of hepatotoxicity[12].

Although clozapine-linked hepatic enzyme changes are usually benign, there are rare case reports of clozapine causing jaundice, hepatic encephalopathy, toxic hepatitis, liver toxicity and fatal acute fulminant liver failure (*Table 10.4.2*). In general, liver function tests showing transaminase values of three times the normal level should warrant enough concern to provoke clinicians either to reduce the dose of clozapine or discontinue completely (particularly if clinical signs of liver damage are evident)[11]. Whether to re-challenge with clozapine following liver toxicity is contentious. There are many case reports where a cautious re-introduction of clozapine, with increased monitoring, was successful once the liver enzymes had returned to normal (*Table 10.4.2*). This however, must be balanced against the severity and symptoms of the liver impairment. In all patients initiated on clozapine, LFTs should be taken at baseline and repeated at least yearly or earlier if clinically indicated[25].

Summary

- Clozapine is extensively eliminated by hepatic mechanisms and liver dysfunction (especially with cirrhosis) is likely significantly to increase clozapine levels.
- In those with liver impairment, common adverse reactions such as constipation and sedation can precipitate hepatic encephalopathy so patients should be actively monitored and treated.
- Clozapine commonly increases liver function tests, usually in the first six weeks of treatment. This increase is largely transient and asymptomatic.
- There are however, rare reports of toxic hepatitis and liver failure associated with clozapine, so any liver enzyme elevated beyond three times the normal level should prompt a dose reduction or discontinuation of clozapine.
- Liver function tests should be routinely monitored before starting clozapine and repeated at least annually or earlier if clinically indicated.

Table 10.4.2: Case reports of liver toxicity associated with clozapine

Author	Age/sex	Daily dose of clozapine	Duration of clozapine treatment	Symptoms/comments
Keane et al, 2009[13]	Case 1. 52, female Case 2. 33, female	1. 100mg 2. 350mg	1. 7 days 2. 5 weeks	1. Symptoms included abdominal pain, generalised malaise. LFTs at peak were ALT 308 IU/L, AST 119 IU/L, GGT 78 IU/L. Clozapine was stopped and LFTs normalised over 4 weeks. Clozapine was re-challenged and LFTs began to elevate again. Clozapine was eventually discontinued at the patient's request 2. LFTs demonstrated a transient rise in AST and ALT which resolved on continued clozapine use
Fong et al, 2005[14]	55, female	200mg	31 days	She developed an itchy urticarial rash, fever, eosinophilia and marked elevation in multiple LFTs (e.g. the ALT was 595 IU/L, normal range <58 IU/L). Clozapine was stopped immediately and the skin rash resolved by day 38 and the LFTs by day 62
Erdogan et al, 2004[15]	27, male	—	2 weeks	Routine monitoring uncovered raised LFTs (AST 111 IU/L, ALT 151 IU/L). Clozapine was discontinued and after 10 days liver enzymes returned to normal. Clozapine was re-introduced and, although LFTs increased again, this resolved over time following a dose reduction
Panagiotis, 1999	30, male	300mg	4 weeks	Presented with a grand mal attack and elevated LFTs. The AST = 116 IU/L, ALT 215 IU/L, GGT 167. Clozapine was discontinued. The patient outcome was not reported
Thompson et al, 1999[17]	48, male	150mg	2 weeks	Symptoms included nausea, anorexia, jaundice and right upper quadrant discomfort. LFTs were raised to ALT 100 IU/L, AST 56IU/L, ALP 257 IU/L. Clozapine was discontinued and LFTs returned to normal over 2 weeks. Obstructive hepatitis secondary to cholelithiasis was diagnosed

Table 10.4.2: Case reports of liver toxicity associated with clozapine *continued*

Author	Age/sex	Daily dose of clozapine	Duration of clozapine treatment	Symptoms/comments
MacFarlane et al, 1997[18]	39, male	350mg	8 weeks	Complaints included nausea, vomiting, abdominal pain and dizziness. He was noted to be extremely jaundiced and had ascites. His total bilirubin was 251 µmol/L, alkaline phosphatise 290 U/L, ALT 1375 U/L and albumin 34 g/L. Despite these symptoms clozapine was continued for a further seven days. He consequently developed grade 2 hepatic encephalo-pathy and despite extensive treatment and investigations died three days later of acute oliguric renal failure and pulmonary oedema. Clozapine was considered the most likely cause of the liver failure
Markowitz et al, 1997[19]	Case 1. 27, male Case 2. 49, male	1. 400mg 2. 300mg	1. 5 weeks 2. 4 weeks	1. No symptoms were reported but LFTs increased to AST 674 IU/L, ALT 1325 IU/L, ALP 144 IU/L, GGT 98 IU/L. Clozapine was discontinued and LFTs normalised over three weeks. On clozapine re-challenge LFTs, AST and ALT began rising again which precipitated clozapine to be withdrawn 2. Presented with persistent diarrhoea. LFTs were increased to ALT 133 IU/L, AST 102 IU/L, ALP 125 IU/L.Clozapine was discontinued and LFTs returned to normal over seven days Both cases also developed eosinophilia
Wirshing et al, 1997[20]	—, female	175mg	6 weeks	She also received semi-sodium valproate. Symptoms included severe, unrousable sedation, asterixis, tender hepatomegaly and mild ascites. ALT= 1525 IU/L, AST=410 IU/L. A diagnosis of hepatic encephalopathy was made and both the clozapine and semi-sodium valproate were stopped. LFTs returned to normal over 3 weeks and clozapine monotherapy was re-introduced

Table 10.4.2: Case reports of liver toxicity associated with clozapine *continued*

Author	Age/sex	Daily dose of clozapine	Duration of clozapine treatment	Symptoms/comments
Worrall et al, 1995[21]	30, female	250mg	14 days	The patient was also hepatitis C seropositive. LFTs were AST = 133IU/L, ALT 424 IU/L. After a dose reduction the LFTs returned to normal over 8 weeks
Thatcher et al, 1995[22]	35, male	300mg	32 days	Symptoms included a pruritic rash, angioedema, joint pain, chills, nausea, fatigue, abdominal pain and diarrhoea. LFT results included ALT 719 U/L and AST 200 U/L. All medication was discontinued and transaminase levels returned to normal over 4–5 weeks
Eggert et al, 1994[23]	40, male	500mg	8 weeks	Asymptomatic but LFTs were AST 177 IU/L, ALT 594 IU/L and ALP 167 IU/L. Clozapine was discontinued and LFTs returned to normal over 30 days. Clozapine was cautiously and successfully re-challenged
Kellner et al, 1993[24]	44, female	400mg	5 weeks	Dramatic increase in LFTs noted at 5 weeks, ALT 675 U/L and AST 369 U/L. Eosinophilia developed. No other symptoms are reported and complete recovery of liver enzymes occurred after four weeks of stopping clozapine

— = not reported; LFT = liver function tests; ALT = alanine aminotransferase (normal values = 10–40 IU/L); AST = aspartate aminotransferase (normal ranges 10–40 IU/L); ALP = alkaline phosphatase (normal values -); GGT = gamma-glutamyl transferase (normal values -0–35 IU/L)

Further reading

Verbeeck R. Pharmacokinetics and dosage adjustments in patients with hepatic dysfunction. *Eur J Clin Pharmacol* 2008; **64:** 1147–61

References

1. Verbeeck R. Pharmacokinetics and dosage adjustments in patients with hepatic dysfunction. *Eur J Clin Pharmacol* 2008; **64:** 1147–61

2. Clozaril specific product characteristics (SPC). Novartis. Available at: www.medicines.org.uk (accessed 12 October 2012).

3. Schaber G, Stevens I, Gaertner H, Dietz K, Breyer-Pfaff U. Pharmacokinetics of clozapine and its metabolites in psychiatric patients: plasma protein binding and renal clearance. *Br J Pharmacol* 1998; **46:** 453–9

4. Morgan D, McLean A. Clinical pharmacokinetics and pharmacodynamics considerations in patients with liver disease. *Clin Pharmacokinet* 1995; **29:** 370–91

5. Jann M, Grimsley S, Gray E, Chang Wen-Ho. Pharmacokinetics and pharmacodynamics of clozapine. *Clin Pharmacokinet* 1993; **24:** 161–76

6. Durand F, Valla D. Assessment of the prognosis of cirrhosis: Child-Pugh versus MELD. *J Hepatol* 2005; **42:** s100–s107

7. Riordan S, Williams R. Treatment of hepatic encephalopathy. *N Engl J Med* 1997; **337:** 473–9

8. Gaertner I, Altendorf K, Batra A, Gaertner H. Relevance of liver enzyme elevations with four different neuroleptics: A retrospective review of 7,263 treatment courses. *J Clin Psychopharmacol* 2001; **21:** 215–22

9. Atasoy N, Erdogan A, Yalug I, Ozturk U, Konuk N, Atik L, et al. A review of liver function tests during treatment with atypical antipsychotic drugs: A chart review study. *Prog Neuropsychopharmacol Biol Psychiatry* 2007; **31:** 1255–60

10. Hummer M, Kurz M, Kurzthaler I, Oberbauer H, Miller C, Fleischhacker W. Hepatotoxicity of clozapine. *J Clin Psychopharmacol* 1997; **17:** 314–17

11. Kaplowitz N. Drug-induced liver disorders. Implication for drug development and regulation. *Drug Safety* 2001; **24:** 483–90

12. Grattagliano I, Bonfrate L, Diogo C, Wang H, Wang D, Portincasa P. Biochemical mechanisms in drug-induced liver injury: Certainties and doubts. *World J Gastroenterol* 2009; **15:** 486–76

13. Keane S, Lane A, Larkin T, Clarke M. Management of clozapine-related hepatotoxicity. *J Clin Psychopharmacol* 2009; **29:** 606–7

14. Fong S, Yeung K, Tosh J, Wing Y. Clozapine-induced toxic hepatitis with skin rash. *J Psychopharmacol* 2005; **19:** 107

15. Erdogan A, Kocabasoglu N, Yalug, I, Ozbay G, Senturk H. Management of marked liver enzyme increased during clozapine treatment: A case report and review of the literature. *Int J Psychiatry Med* 2004; **34:** 83–9

16. Panagiotis B. Grand Mal seizures with liver toxicity in a case of clozapine treatment. *J Neuropsychiatry Clin Neurosci* 1999; **11:** 117–18

17. Thompson J, Chengappa K, Good C, Baker R, Kiewe R, Bezner J, et al. Hepatitis, hyperglycemia, pleural effusion, eosinophilia, hematuria and protinuria occurring early in clozapine treatment. *Int Clin Psychopharmacol* 1998; **13:** 95–8

18. MacFarlane B, Davies S, Mannan K, Sarsam R, Pariente D Dooley J. Fatal acute fulminant liver failure due to clozapine: A case report and review of clozapine-induced hepatotoxicity. *Gastroenterology* 1997; **112:** 1707–9

19. Markowitz J, Grinberg R, Jackson C. Marked liver enzyme elevations with clozapine. *J Clin Psychopharmacol* 1997; **17:** 70–1

20. Wirshing W, Ames D, Bisheff S, Pierre J, Mendoza A, Sun A. Hepatic encephalopathy associated with combined clozapine and divalproex. *J Clin Psychopharmacol* 1997; **17:** 120–1

21. Worrall R, Wilson A, Cullen M. Dystonia and drug-induced hepatitis in a patient treated with clozapine. *Am J Psychiatry* 152; **4:** 647–8

22. Tatcher G, Cates M, Bair B. Clozapine-induced Toxic Hepatitis. *Am J Psychiatry* 1995; **152:** 296–7
23. Eggert A, Crismon M, Dorson P, Taylor R. Clozapine re-challenge after marked liver enzyme elevation. *J Clin Psychopharmacol* 1994; **14:** 425–6
24. Kellner M, Wiedemann K, Krieg J, Berg P. Toxic hepatitis by clozapine treatment. *Am J Psychiatry* 1993; **150:** 985–6
25. Taylor D, Paton C, Kapur S. *The Maudsley Prescribing guidelines.* 11th edition: Chichester: Wiley-Blackwell: 2012

10.5: The elderly

The complex process of aging has profound effects on the pharmacokinetic and pharmacodynamic properties of drugs such as clozapine (*Figure 10.5.1*). The risk of severe adverse effects and drug toxicity increase with age because of the decline in function of multiple systems. In addition, as the prevalence of comorbid diseases increases the potential for polypharmacy, so the risk of drug interactions rises. Prescribing clozapine in the elderly poses specific problems and requires significant caution.

Figure 10.5.1: Factors in aging which may modify the pharmacokinetic and dynamic properties of clozapine[1,2]
General body systems:
Weight loss and frailty (increasing plasma concentrations and adverse reactions)
Multiple system diseases (concurrent medication = increased risk of interactions)
Reduction in dopaminergic and cholinergic neurones (increased risk of concurrent movement disorders and anticholinergic drug effects)
Reduction in homeostatic mechanisms (increased risk of postural hypotension and falls)
Declining immune system (increased susceptibility for infections)
Increased body fat (increased volume of distribution and half-life)
Decreased serum albumin (increased free fraction in plasma)
Individual organ changes:
Decreased gastrointestinal motility (slower absorption and increased risk of constipation)
Decreased renal blood flow and glomerular filtration rate (reduced renal elimination)
Reduced hepatic mass and blood flow (reduced first pass metabolism and slower cytochrome metabolism)
Reduced cardiac output (increased susceptibility to postural hypotension and falls)

While aging can affect clozapine pharmacokinetics in many ways, the most important change is the decline in renal and liver function. Renal blood flow reduces by approximately 1% per year after the age of 40, and this, combined with other factors, causes a reduction in glomerular filtration by 25–50% between the ages of 20 and 90[2]. The estimated glomerular filtration rate (eGFR) is recommended as an appropriate tool to track renal function in the elderly (*Chapter 10.3*)[1]. Although clozapine may not accumulate in those with only mild or moderate renal impairment, it has many adverse reactions which can worsen renal impairment (diabetes, nocturnal enuresis, urinary retention, sedation and hypotension).

Changes to liver functioning take various forms in the elderly. Liver blood flow reduces by approximately 40%, total liver size decreases by 25–30%, bile flow is reduced and consequently production of blood proteins, lipids and glucose can be affected[2]. Metabolising capacity, through phase I cytochrome P450 enzymes, does not appear to be affected by aging (except when cirrhosis is present), but as blood flow is reduced the rate of metabolism may be affected[2]. Clozapine may therefore accumulate because of slower metabolism and increased free blood levels may give rise to more severe adverse effects. Those with cirrhosis or clinical signs of liver damage may be particularly at risk. It is also important to remember that clozapine commonly causes a transient increase in liver enzymes, and adverse effects such as sedation and constipation can cause complications in people with liver impairment (*Chapter 10.4*).

Pharmacodynamic changes in aging

Age-related effects on receptor number, signal transduction and homeostatic mechanisms[2] can also reduce the tolerability of clozapine. For example, the elderly commonly have a reduction in cholinergic neurones and receptors and this may be involved in cognitive decline[3]. Clozapine, with prominent anticholinergic properties, may further impair cognition and cause confusion in old age[3]. Homeostatic functions, such as the regulation of arterial blood pressure can take longer to balance in the elderly so drugs with prominent α_1-adrenoceptor blockade, such as clozapine, can worsen orthostatic hypotension and consequently cause syncope and falls[2,4].

Clozapine for schizophrenia in later life

There are no large, randomised, placebo controlled studies of clozapine use in elderly patients with schizophrenia. However for treatment-resistant schizophrenia, clozapine is uniquely effective, and so for those elderly patients who are unresponsive to other antipsychotics clozapine may be appropriate[5]. *Table 10.5.1* outlines the evidence base supporting the use of clozapine in elderly patients with psychotic disorders and the reported outcomes. In summary, there are over 500 reports of using clozapine in elderly people with schizophrenia (or similar conditions), and the vast majority of data suggest it is effective, although with a number of adverse effects. The most commonly used dose in these reports is between 100 and 300mg per day. Frequent adverse effects reported in the elderly are dizziness, sedation, postural hypotension and hypersalivation.
Of concern is that some authors report a higher risk of agranulocytosis in older patients[9,10,12]

Table 10.5.1: The evidence base supporting clozapine use for schizophrenia and related disorders in the elderly (– = unclear or not reported)

Author (type of study)	Number of patients	Age range	Doses range per day (mean)	Duration of treatment (mean)	Diagnosis	Comment
Schizophrenia or psychotic disorders						
Snowdon et al, 2011[6] (case series)	16	65–76 (72)	100-600mg (330mg)	2 months–9 years	Mostly chronic schizophrenia	13 /16 reported some or much improvement. 14/16 experienced side-effects such as postural hypotension, sedation, hypersalivation, ataxia
O'Connor et al, 2010[7] (retrospective review)	75	65–89 (74.2)	25–800mg (296mg)	4–132 months	Mostly treatment-resistant schizophrenia (71%)	Effectiveness was not rated. 37 (49%) had discontinued treatment by the time of the review, 14 because of death (1 possibly related to clozapine), 12 due to adverse effects and 8 due to patient choice. The three most common adverse effects were sedation, hypersalivation and constipation
Howanitz et al, 1999[8] (double blind comparison study with chlorpromazine)	24 on clozapine	- (65)	- (300mg)	12 weeks	Schizophrenia	Clozapine numerically more effective than chlorpromazine. Both groups had equal number of side-effects and all patients reported at least one side-effect
Barak et al, 1999[9] (literature review)	139	65–82	6.25–600mg (134.5mg)	–	Mixed	Efficacy was reported as significant in the majority of cases who had appropriate durations of treatment. 11.5% experienced adverse effects with the three most common being hypersalivation, leucopenia and orthostatic hypotension, 5% experienced haematological disturbances
Sajatovic et al, 1998[10] (naturalistic review)	329	55–86 (63.4)	12.5–900mg (310mg)	2–1,379 days (278 days)	Treat refractory, or treatment intolerant psychosis	Improvement in positive symptoms was demonstrated. The age group 55–64 showed the greatest improvement.

Table 10.5.1: The evidence base supporting clozapine use for schizophrenia and related disorders in the elderly *continued*

Author (type of study)	Number of patients	Age range	Doses range per day (mean)	Duration of treatment (mean)	Diagnosis	Comment
Sajatovic et al, 1998[10] (naturalistic review), *continued*	329	55–86 (63.4)	12.5–900mg (310mg)	2–1,379 days (278 days)	Treat refractory, or treatment intolerant psychosis	The most common adverse reactions were sedation (11.2%), haematologic side-effects (6.5%), hypotension and tachycardia (5.6%)
Sajatovic et al 1997[11] (open label trial)	10	65–76 (70.6)	12.5–375mg (204mg)	13–2417 days (430 days)	Primary psychotic disorders	7/10 had a clinical improvement. The mean improvement on BPRS was 22%. Side-effects included sedation (3/10), drooling (4/10), and normal sinus tachycardia (3/10)
Herst et al, 1997[12] (case reports)	5	63–79 (68.6)	100–250mg (120mg)		Schizophrenia/ schizoaffective	2/5 demonstrated a marked improvement, 3/5 had an initial improvement which appeared to wear off. 4/5 experienced an adverse reaction
Pitner et al, 1995[13] (case reports)	4	68–83	6.25–37.5mg		Refractory psychosis (three also had dementia)	Two experienced a clinical benefit, all four experienced adverse effects including falls, bradycardia and delirium
Salzman et al, 1995[14] (retrospective review)	20	65–84 (72)	75–350mg (210mg)	2–14 months	Behavioral disruption secondary to psychosis	The authors report a clear and significant improvement in all patients (although no formal rating scales were used). Adverse effects were 12/20 reported sedation, 4/20 reported breathing problems, 3/20 reported pneumonia and 3/20 reported leukopenia
Chengappa et al, 1995[15] (retrospective review)	12	61–82 (68.8)	25–300mg (-)	7days–8 months	Chronic schizophrenia	7/12 showed some improvement. 10/12 reported a notable side-effect. Most common side-effects were dizziness, postural hypotension, and sedation. Authors report clozapine was tolerated better when clinician used a slower initial titration

Clozapine for drug-induced psychosis in Parkinson's disease

Psychosis in Parkinson's disease is generally (but not always) associated with the medication used to treat movement disorders[16]. Treatment of psychosis usually begins with a reduction in the dose of the presumed causative medication (such as anticholinergics or dopamine agonists), but this action needs to be weighed against the likelihood of worsening motor functioning[16]. Clozapine has three, randomised, placebo-controlled trials supporting its use in psychosis in Parkinson's disease (*Table 10.5.2*). It is considered to be more effective and less likely to cause motor deterioration than risperidone[17], olanzapine[18] and quetiapine[19] but, it is usually considered second line after other atypical antipsychotics because of the necessary associated monitoring and extensive adverse effects[20]. Where clozapine is used it is often effective at very low doses (between 6.25–50mg per day), usually works within a week and may improve tremor even in those whose symptoms have been resistant to other treatments[16]. The doses at which clozapine is effective suggest a different pharmacological mechanism from that in schizophrenia. The main adverse effects seen when used in Parkinson's disease are sedation, orthostatic hypotension and hypersalivation[16]. Clozapine has been shown to be effective in the treatment of Parkinson's disease psychosis for up to five years[21]. As is the case with schizophrenia, clozapine is likely to be underutilised in Parkinson's disease psychosis[16].

Clozapine for other disorders

The evidence base for using clozapine in other mental disorders in the elderly is limited to case series or case reports (*Table 10.5.3*). There is also no evidence to support clozapine use in the very old (>85 years).

Plasma levels of clozapine in the elderly

Although results of studies on plasma clozapine concentrations and age have been inconsistent, the most recent and largest studies point to an age-related increase in levels (+4% with every five years after 40 years)[29]. Older female patients would appear to be at the greatest risk of a higher plasma concentration[29,30], with the changes being most likely due to reduced clearance and altered metabolic capacity[30].

Covert administration

Concealing medication in food or drink ('covert administration') should only be considered in exceptional circumstances. National guidelines exist to prevent the unlawful and inappropriate administration of medication in this way[31,32]. Covert administration should be considered only where there is full agreement of all multidisciplinary team members, family and carers and only after other options have been fully exhausted[33]. Clozapine is widely available as a liquid (in the UK as Denzapine® 50mg/ml oral suspension)[34] and this may prove a useful option in those who have difficulty swallowing or who retain the tablet in their mouth for later disposal. There is no literature investigating the stability of crushed clozapine in food or drink[35], although a survey conducted in 1999 suggested it is occasionally done in practice[36]. Given the ready availability of the liquid preparation, tablet crushing is unnecessary. A clozapine oral disintegrating tablet is also available in some countries and may be another useful option.

Table 10.5.2: RCTs supporting clozapine use in Parkinson's disease

Author (type of study)	Number of patients	Age range	Doses range per day (mean)	Duration of treatment (mean)	Diagnosis	Comment
Pollak et al, 2004[22] (RCT)	32 on clozapine	(71.2)	12.5–50mg (35.8mg)	4 weeks followed by a 12-week open trial	Drug induced psychosis in Parkinson's disease	From the first week of treatment clozapine proved more effective than placebo. The maximum improvement was seen after 2–3 months of clozapine use. A relapse in symptoms was observed in 19/25 patients who at the end of the trial were withdrawn from clozapine. Somnolence (53%), worsening of Parkinson's symptoms (21.8%), postural hypotension (19%) and respiratory infections (16%) were the most common adverse effects during the first four weeks
Durif et al, 2004[23] (RCT)	26 on clozapine	61–67	(39.4mg)	10 weeks	Levodopa-induced dyskinesias (LID)	LID score was significantly reduced with clozapine and there was a reduction in 'on' periods with LID. 3/26 in the clozapine group developed eosinophilia which resolved on discontinuation
The Parkinson Study group, 1999[24] (RCT)	30 on clozapine	(72)	6.25–50mg (24.7mg)	14 months	Drug-induced psychosis in Parkinson's disease	Improvements favouring clozapine were seen in all measures (CGI, BPRS, SAPS). 13/60 showed complete remission. There was also a significantly beneficial effect in tremor in the clozapine group.

Table 10.5.2: RCTs supporting clozapine use in Parkinson's disease *continued*

Author (type of study)	Number of patients	Age range	Doses range per day (mean)	Duration of treatment (mean)	Diagnosis	Comment
The Parkinson Study group, 1999[24] (RCT) *continued*	30 on clozapine	(72)	6.25–50mg (24.7mg)	14 months	Drug-induced psychosis in Parkinson's disease	No impairment in cognition was measured. Weight gain and tachycardia were reported more than placebo
The French Clozapine Parkinson Study Group, 1999[25] (double blind-placebo controlled trial)	32 on clozapine	(72)	6.25–50mg (36mg)	4 weeks	Drug-induced psychosis in Parkinson's disease	Significant changes in CGI score and PANNS positive sub-score in favour of clozapine was noted from the first week. 7/32 reported worsening of parkinsonism (usually mild or transient). Somnolence was also more frequently reported in the clozapine group

Table 10.5.3: Evidence base supporting clozapine use in other disorders in the elderly

Author (type of study)	Number of patients	Age range	Doses range per day (mean)	Duration of treatment (mean)	Diagnosis	Comment
Lee et al, 2007[26] (retrospective review)	16	— (66.8)	- (34.2mg)	- (34.5 days)	Agitation in dementia (8 had Parkinson's disease)	10/16 (62.5%) were rated as much improved. MMSE scores did not change. Adverse effects included drooling (5 reports), sedation (5 reports), constipation (1 report) and delirium (3 reports)
Srinivasan, 1999[27] (case reports)	4	—	12.5–50mg (-)	2–6 months (–)	Behavioral problems in dementia	All four responded, one report of sedation. Limited details
Shulam et al, 1997[28] (case reports)	3	70–74	25–112.5mg	(11 months)	Bipolar I disorder (mania with psychotic features)	All 3 greatly improved. One report of myoclonus which resolved on lowering clozapine dose, one report of sedation, hypotension and thrombocytopenia which improved on reducing the dose

Conclusion

Despite expected poor tolerability and the relatively limited evidence base, clozapine appears to be an acceptable and useful choice for old age psychiatrists[37] where other antipsychotics have failed in both schizophrenia and drug-induced psychosis in Parkinson's disease. There is little evidence to support clozapine use in other disorders in old age and there is no evidence of use in the very old (above 85 years).

In the authors' clinical opinion, where clozapine is considered appropriate, it would be better to start extremely slowly in the elderly (e.g. 6.25mg a day), increase more slowly than in adults (e.g. 6.25–12.5mg per day) and aim for a lower maintenance dose, 100–300mg per day for schizophrenia and 6.25–50mg per day in Parkinson's disease.

Summary

- Elderly patients are more prone to drug adverse effects, toxicity and interactions than younger patients.
- Although poorly tolerated, clozapine appears an appropriate choice in elderly patients with treatment-resistant schizophrenia or drug-induced psychosis in Parkinson's disease.
- Where clozapine is appropriate, start extremely slowly in the elderly (e.g. 6.25mg a day), increase slower than in younger adults (e.g. 6.25–12.5mg per day) and aim for a lower maintenance dose: 100–300mg per day for schizophrenia and 6.25–50mg per day in Parkinson's disease.
- There is no robust data supporting clozapine in other disorders in old age and no evidence supporting its use in the very old.

Further reading

Gareri P, De Fazio P, Russo E, Marigliano N, De Fazia S, De Sarro G. The safety of clozapine in the elderly. *Expert Opinion Drug Safety* 2008; **7:** 525–38

References

1. Klotz U. Pharmacokinetic and drug metabolism in the elderly. *Drug Metab Rev* 2009; **41:** 67–76
2. Turnheim K. When drug therapy gets old: pharmacokinetic and pharmacodynamics in the elderly. *Exp Gerontol* 2003; **38:** 843–53
3. Mintzer J. Anticholinergic side-effects of drugs in elderly people. *J Royal Soc Med* 2000; **93:** 457–62
4. Gareri P, De Fazio P, Russo E, Marigliano N, De Fazia S, De Sarro G. The safety of clozapine in the elderly. *Expert Opinion Drug Safety* 2008; **7:** 525–38
5. Sajatovic M, Madhusoodanam S, Buckley P. Schizophrenia in the elderly. Guidelines for management. *CNS Drugs* 2000; **13:** 103–15

6. Snowdon J, Halliday G. A study of the use of clozapine in old age psychiatry. *Int Clin Psychopharmacol* 2011; **26:** 232–5
7. O'Connor D, Sierakowski C, Chin L, Singh D. The safety and tolerability of clozapine in aged patients: A retrospective clinical file review. *World Biol Psychiatry* 2010; **11:** 788–91
8. Howanitz E, Pardo M, Smelson D, Engelhart C, Eisenstein N, Losonczy M. The efficacy and safety of clozapine versus chlorpromazine in geriatric schizophrenia. *J Clin Psychiatry* 1999; **60:** 41–4
9. Barak Y, Wittenberg N, Naor S, Kutzuk D, Weizman A. Clozapine in elderly psychiatric patients: tolerability, safety and efficacy. *Compre Psychiatry* 1999; **40:** 320–5
10. Sajatovic M, Ramirez L, Garver D, Thompson P, Ripper G, Lehmann L. clozapine therapy for older veterans. *Psychiatr Serv* 1998; **49:** 340–4
11. Sajatovic M, Jaskiw G, Konicki E, Jurjus G, Kwon K, Ramirez L. Outcome of clozapine therapy for elderly patients with refractory primary psychosis. *Int J Geriatr Psychiatry* 1997; **12:** 553–8
12. Herst L, Powell G. Is clozapine safe in the elderly. *Aust N Z J Psychiatry* 1997; **31:** 411–17
13. Pitner J, Mintzer J, Pennypacker L, Jackson C. Efficacy and adverse effects of clozapine in four elderly psychotic patients. *J Clin Psychiatry* 1995; **56:** 180–5
14. Salzman C, Vaccaro B, Lieff J, Weiner A. Clozapine in older patients with psychosis and behavioral disruption. *Am J Geriatr Psychiatry* 1995; **3:** 26–33
15. Chengappa K, Baker R, Kreinbrook S, Adair D. Clozapine use in female geriatric patients with psychosis. *J Geriatr Psychiatry Neurol* 1995; **8:** 12–15
16. Friedman J. Parkinson's disease psychosis 2010: a review article. *Parkinsonism Relat Disord* 2010; **16:** 553–60.
17. Ellis T, Cudkowicz M, Sexton P, Growdon J. Clozapine and risperidone treatment of psychosis in Parkinson's disease. *J Neuropsychiatry Clin Neurosci* 2000; **12:** 364–9
18. Friedman J, Goldstein S, Jacques C. Substituting clozapine for olanzapine in psychiatrically stable Parkinson's disease patients: results of an open label pilot study. *Clin Neuropharmacol* 1998; **21:** 285–8
19. Merims D, Balas M, Peretz C, Shabtai H, Giladi N. Rater-blinded, prospective comparison: Quetiapine versus clozapine for Parkinson's disease psychosis. *Clin Neuropharmacol* 2006; **29:** 331–7
20. National Institute for Health and Clinical Excellence. *Parkinson's Disease: Diagnosis and management in primary and secondary care. Clinical Guideline 35.* Available at: http://www.nice.org.uk . 2006. (accessed November 2012)
21. Klein C, Gordon J, Pollak L, Rabey J. Clozapine in Parkinson's disease psychosis: 5-year follow up review. *Clin Neuropharmacol* 2003; **26:** 8–11
22. Pollak P, Tison F, Rascol O, Destée A, Péré J, Senard J, et al. Clozapine in drug induced psychosis in Parkinson's disease : a randomised, placebo controlled study with open label follow up. *J Neurol Neurosurg Psychiatry* 2004; **75:** 689–95
23. Durif F, Debilly B, Galitzky M, Morand D, Viallet F, Borg M, et al. Clozapine improves dyskinesias in Parkinson disease. A double-blind, placebo-controlled study. *Neurology* 2004; **62:** 381–8
24. The Parkinson Study Group. Low-dose clozapine for the treatment of drug-induced psychosis in Parkinson's disease. *N Engl J Med* 1999; **340:** 757–63
25. The French Clozapine Parkinson Study Group. Clozapine in drug-induced psychosis in Parkinson's disease. *Lancet* 1999; **353:** 2041–2

26. Lee H, Hanner J, Yokley J, Appleby B, Hurowitz L, Lyketsos C. Clozapine for treatment-resistant agitation in dementia. *J Geriatr Psychiatry Neurol* 2007; **20:** 178–82
27. Srinivasan T. Clozapine for psychotic and behavioral problems in dementia. *Indian J Psychiatry* 1999; **41:** 171
28. Shulman R, Singh A, Shulam K. Treatment of elderly institutionalized bipolar patients with clozapine. *Psychopharmacol Bull* 1997; **33:** 113–18
29. Rostami-Hodjegan A, Amin A, Spencer E, Lennard M, Tucker G, Flannagan R. Influence of dose, cigarette smoking, age, sex and metabolic activity on plasma clozapine concentrations: A predictive model and nomograms to aid clozapine dose adjustments and to assess compliance in individual patients. *J Clin Psychopharmacol* 2004; **24:** 70–8
30. Ismail Z, Wessels A, Uchida H, Ng W, Mamo D, Rajji T, et al. Age and sex impact clozapine plasma level concentrations in inpatients and outpatients with schizophrenia. *Am J Geriatr Psychiatry* 2012; **20:** 53–60
31. Nursing and Midwifery Council. Covert administration of medicines — disguising medicines in food and drink. 2007. Available at: http://www.nmc-uk.org.uk
32. Royal College of Psychiatrists. College statement on covert administration of medicines. *Psychiatric Bull* 2004; **28:** 385–6
33. Mental Welfare Commission for Scotland. Covert medication. Legal and Practice guidelines. November 2006. Available at: www.mwcscot.org.uk (accessed November 2012)
34. Denzapine 50mg/ml oral suspension specific product characteristics (SPC). Genus. Available at: www.medicines.org.uk (accessed 15th November 2012)
35. Clozaril Patient Monitoring Service (CPMS). Personal communication. 15 November 2012
36. Pereira S, Beer D, Paton C. Enforcing treatment with clozapine: A survey of views and practice. *Psychiatr Bull* 1999; **23:** 342–5
37. Paranthaman R, Baldwin R. Survey of clozapine use by consultant old age psychiatrists. *Psychiatr Bull* 2006; **30:** 410–12

10.6: Children and adolescents

The use of clozapine in children and adolescents is a contentious issue. On one hand sits the concern of exposing a young person with a developing brain to a potentially dangerous drug. Countering this are the severe and enduring symptoms of schizophrenia with which children can present and the need to effectively tackle them to prevent a poor lifetime outcome. Most experts, however, agree that clozapine, with very close monitoring for adverse events, is appropriate in youths with schizophrenia who do not respond to other antipsychotics[1,2].

Schizophrenia in children and adolescents

Childhood-onset or prepubertal schizophrenia (onset of symptoms before 13 years) is a rare but severe form of the disorder which is often treatment resistant[3]. Early onset schizophrenia (onset of symptoms before 18 years) is relatively more common and accounts for approximately 12–33% of individuals with schizophrenia[4]. In both conditions an insidious onset, premorbid abnormalities and a high rate of negative symptoms are frequent and predict a poorer long-term outcome[3]. Between 50 and 90% of children presenting with schizophrenia continue to have symptoms into adolescence and adulthood, and those with symptoms before the age of 10 have the worst prognosis[3].

There are a number of clinical trials supporting antipsychotics in children and adolescents with schizophrenia[3]. Clozapine has been investigated in three RCTs (*Table 10.6.1*) in those who are either intolerant or unresponsive to at least two other antipsychotics. These studies have demonstrated greater improvements in symptoms than with both olanzapine and haloperidol, but clozapine is associated with a greater burden of adverse events, most notably seizures and neutropenia.

The National Institute for Health and Clinical Excellence (NICE) pooled data from the three RCTs and, although acknowledging the limitations of the studies, similarly concluded that clozapine resulted in moderately better symptom control than olanzapine or haloperidol[8]. The NICE recommendations were:

> *Offer clozapine to children and young people whose illness has not responded adequately to pharmacological treatment despite the sequential use of adequate doses of at least two different antipsychotic drugs.*

Based on adult studies where clozapine was augmented with another antipsychotic, NICE also suggest[8]:

> *For children and young people whose illness has not responded adequately to clozapine at an optimised dose, consider a multidisciplinary review, and*

recommendation (including measuring therapeutic drug levels) before adding a second antipsychotic to augment treatment with clozapine. An adequate trial of such an augmentation may need to be up to 8–10 weeks. Choose a drug that does not compound the common side-effects of clozapine.

Table 10.6.1: RCTs supporting clozapine use in childhood-onset schizophrenia

Author (type of study)	Number of patients	Age range, years (mean)	Doses range per day (mean)	Duration of treatment (mean)	Diagnosis	Comment
Kumra et al, 2008[5] (RCT comparison with 'high dose' olanzapine)	18 on clozapine	10–18 (15.6)	50–700mg (403.1mg)	12 weeks	Early onset schizophrenia or schizoaffective disorder refractory to two previous antipsychotic trials	Significantly more (P=0.038) clozapine-treated patients (66%) met response criteria than the olanzapine group (33%). 5 patients (one on olanzapine, 4 on clozapine) experienced 'serious' adverse effects
Shaw et al, 2006[6] (RCT comparison with olanzapine)	12 on clozapine	7–16 (12.3)	150–500mg (327mg)	8 weeks with a 2-year follow-up	Childhood-onset schizophrenia resistant to at least 2 antipsychotics	The change in symptom score (SANS, CGI-S, SAPS) was consistently greater for clozapine (vs. olanzapine) and clozapine was associated with large to moderate treatment effect sizes. Clozapine was associated with more adverse effects such as tachycardia, hypertension and enuresis
Kumra et al, 1996[7] (RCT comparison with haloperidol)	10 on clozapine	6–18 (14)	125–525mg (239mg)	6 weeks followed by a 2-year monthly telephone follow-up	Schizophrenia with onset by age 12, intolerant or unresponsive to 2 different antipsychotics	Clozapine was superior to haloperidol on all measures of psychosis (P=0.04-0.002). The clozapine group experienced more reports of drowsiness and hypersalivation than haloperidol. 5 patients in the clozapine group experienced a drop in neutrophil count and 2 had significant seizure activity

A number of open label and retrospective studies also support clozapine use in early-onset schizophrenia (*Table 10.6.2*). Despite the small samples sizes in these controlled studies, the evidence base supporting clozapine in treatment-resistant early-onset schizophrenia is encouraging. Perhaps the most compelling aspect of these data is the uniformity of findings in respect to clozapine's superiority. The initial doses of clozapine in the literature suggest a slightly slower titration than in the adult population (e.g. starting at 12.5mg per day and increasing by 12.5–25mg every 2–3 days), with the average maintenance dose being between 250 and 350mg per day.

Table 10.6.2: Other clinical trials supporting clozapine use in early-onset schizophrenia

Author (type of study)	Number of patients	Age range, years (mean)	Doses range per day (mean)	Duration of treatment (mean)	Diagnosis	Comment
Kumra et al, 2008[9] (open-label extension study vs. high dose olanzapine)	14 on clozapine	10–18 (15.5)	—	24 weeks	Early onset schizophrenia refractory to two previous antipsychotic trials	A significantly (P=0.001) higher proportion of clozapine patients (86%) remained on treatment compared with the olanzapine group (42%). Weight gain was a major concern in both groups
Kim et al, 2008[10] (retrospective study)	26	7–13 (14.4)	50–475mg (278.8)	Length of follow up 3.6 years ± 2.8 years	Treatment-resistant early-onset schizophrenia	Clozapine significantly decreased the number of hospitalisations per year and this effect persisted throughout the follow-up. Neutropenia occurred in 26.9% of patients but all were maintained and successfully re-challenged with clozapine
Sporn et al, 2007[11] (re-analysis of results from previous studies)	(recruited from the RCTs listed in *Table 10.6.1*, or open label studies)	7–19.1 (13.5) — initial 6 weeks	75–800 (298.2mg) — initial 6 weeks	6 weeks with up to 6 years follow-up	Treatment-resistant childhood-onset schizophrenia	At 6 weeks 39% were considered clozapine responders (≥20% improvement on the BPRS). Improvement continued during follow-up. The most common adverse effects reported were tachycardia, hypersalivation and EEG changes

Table 10.6.2: Other clinical trials supporting clozapine use in early-onset schizophrenia *continued*

Author (type of study)	Number of patients	Age range, years (mean)	Doses range per day (mean)	Duration of treatment (mean)	Diagnosis	Comment
Kranzler et al, 2005[12] (retrospective review — focusing on aggression)	20	- (15.78)	476mg ± 119mg	6 months	Treatment-resistant childhood-onset schizophrenia or schizo-affective disorder	A significant decrease in oral and IM medication used for aggression was demonstrated also with a reduction in seclusion
Turetz et al 199713 (open trial)	11	9-11 (11.3)	200-300 (227.3mg)	16 weeks with 3 year follow up	Treatment resistant childhood-onset schizophrenia	Rating scales reduced in value by 42%-CGI, 70% BPRS and 50%-PANSS indicating significant improvement with clozapine. The majority of the improvement was shown in the first 6 weeks of treatment. Drowsiness, hyper-salivation and EEG changes were the most common adversc reactions reported
Frazier, 1994[14] (open trial)	11	12–17 (14)	125–825mg (370.5mg)	6 weeks	Childhood-onset schizophrenia resistant or intolerant to two previous antipsychotics	Overall there was a 58% improvement in CGI and SAPS scores, from baseline. 82% showed a greater than 30% improvement on baseline BPRS scores. The most common adverse effects were hypersalivation, sedation and weight gain

CGI = Clinical global impression; SPPS = Scale for the Assessment of Positive Symptoms;
BPRS = Brief Psychiatric Rating Scale

Other psychiatric disorders in children and adolescents: the role of clozapine

Studies investigating clozapine use in other psychiatric disorders seen in children and adolescents are limited to case reports or small case series. Masi et al described the therapeutic effect of clozapine in ten adolescents (age range being 12–17-year-olds) inpatients with severe acute mania or mixed episodes. All were resistant to conventional mood stabilisers. Patients were followed up for 12–24 months and all were considered responders, each scoring 1 or 2 on the CGI scale. The mean effective dose of clozapine was 142.5mg per day (range 75–300mg) and the average time to a response of the mood disorder was 15 days[15].

There are three case reports describing clozapine use in adolescents with autism spectrum disorders and severe disruptive behaviour[16] and a brief case series (n=6) on using clozapine for children and adolescents with serious conduct disorders[17]. Until larger controlled trials are conducted, clozapine is not recommended in young people for any diagnosis other than treatment-resistant schizophrenia.

Adverse reactions in children and adolescents

Adverse effects seen with clozapine in children and adolescents are broadly similar to those reported in the adult population. Clozapine is unlikely to increase prolactin or cause movement disorders in the young, but commonly causes weight gain, sedation, hypersalivation and tachycardia. In growing children, body weight is expected to rise so using body mass index and adjusting for age and gender will give a more accurate picture of any weight changes associated with clozapine (*Figure 10.6.1*). Weight gain and obesity (defined in children as BMI ≥95th percentile) are associated with metabolic syndrome (dyslipidaemia, glucose intolerance and hypertension) which, when found in the young, predicts atherosclerosis and vascular disease in early adulthood[18]. In a RCT by Shaw et al, the average weight gain with clozapine over eight weeks was 3.8kg (±6 kg)[6]. Leptin levels have also been shown to increase in young patients with childhood-onset schizophrenia[19]. Hyperleptinaemia has been linked with developing obesity and insulin-resistance, and reflects a loss of hormonal control of appetite and catabolism of fat[19].

Young people exposed to clozapine may also be at a higher risk of developing seizures or having EEG changes than adults[13]. Many experts advocate a baseline EEG, which is repeated around six weeks after clozapine initiation[1]. In addition,

Figure 10.6.1: Measuring body mass index (BMI) in children and adolescents

$$BMI = (\text{weight in kg})/(\text{height in metres})^2$$

Tables and charts of normal values for BMI for age and gender are available at:
www.cdc.gov/growthcharts

A handy online child and adult BMI weight calculator can be found at:
http://www.nhs.uk/Tools/Pages/Healthyweightcalculator.aspx

there are suggestions that neutropenia with clozapine is more common in children and adolescents compared with adults. In a poster abstract by David et al in 2012 (n=87, mean age 13.35 years), moderate neutropenia was reported in 20% of adolescents exposed to clozapine. Younger age, African American ethnicity and male gender were significant risk factors for neutropenia in the young[20].

To help quantify the risks associated with clozapine in children and adolescents, clinicians should investigate the physical health of first-degree relatives and see if this could highlight any potential risks before initiating treatment. History of diabetes dyslipidaemia and obesity would be particularly important in this respect.

Plasma levels in children and adolescents

Although there is some support for dosing clozapine based on plasma levels in children and adolescents[21], the level associated with clinical response in the absence of toxicity has not been established. Plasma clozapine levels appear to be related to the prescribed dose and in 16–17-year-olds, factors such as smoking, clozapine to norclozapine ratio, gender, age and body weight affect clozapine concentrations similarly to adults[21]. In the younger age group (8–15-year-olds), gender and smoking appear less significant[21].

Licensing issues

The manufacturers of clozapine state that the drug is not recommended in children and adolescents under the age of 16 years because the safety and efficacy has not been established[22]. Prescribing for those under 16 therefore becomes 'off label', that is, using a licenced medicine in an unlicensed way. The Royal College of Psychiatrists in the UK provides ten recommendations to consider for such prescribing (*Figure 10.6.2*)[23]. In addition to these recommendations, prescribers should openly discuss the risks and benefits of clozapine with the child, parents or guardians and follow this discussion up with appropriate written advice.

Conclusion

As with the adult population, clozapine is probably underutilised in children and adolescents with treatment-resistant schizophrenia. This may in part be unfamiliarity with clozapine or a concern with the potential adverse reactions and the burden of associated monitoring[24]. Adverse effects appear broadly similar to those seen in adults with the exception of an increased risk of neutropenia, EEG changes and seizures.

Figure 10.6.2: Recommendations for suggested procedure when prescribing medication 'off-label'[23]

1. Check that medicines with a product licence have either had a proper therapeutic trial or been considered, but excluded on clinical grounds (such as contraindications and risk of interactions).
2. Familiarise yourself with the evidence about the proposed drug, including any possible drug interactions and potential adverse effects.
3. If the medicine to be used does not have a substantial evidence-base supporting its use for the proposed indication, or if you are not sufficiently expert in this field, or have particular concerns, obtain the advice of another doctor or specialist pharmacist.
4. Consider the risks and benefits of the proposed treatment. Particular consideration is needed with children, older patients, and in those with impaired insight and judgement. Document this.
5. Give the patient (or his/her relative, when relevant) a full explanation, including the information that the drug will be used outside its product licence. Document this explanation.
6. If agreement from the patient (or his/her relative, when needed) is obtained, document this approval. If a patient is unable to consent to a necessary treatment, note that it has not been possible to obtain consent.
7. Begin a cautious trial of treatment with the medicine. In outpatients, consider sending the patient a copy of any letter sent to his/her general practitioner, summarising why this approach has been adopted.
8. Monitor the patient closely. Continue with full documentation of its effectiveness and tolerance.
9. If the treatment proves unsuccessful, withdraw it, gradually if needed. Document the reason for the withdrawal of treatment, then consider alternatives, using the same process.
10. Consider writing up the case, to add to knowledge about the drug and its use.

Summary

- Clozapine is recommended for childhood-onset schizophrenia or early onset schizophrenia which has failed to respond to at least two other antipsychotics, which have been tried for an adequate time and dose.
- The evidence base for clozapine in other psychiatric disorders is poor, so clozapine cannot be recommended for other childhood conditions.
- Adverse reactions in the young appear broadly similar to those seen in adults, with the exception that EEG changes and seizures appear more frequent.
- A baseline EEG, which is repeated six weeks into clozapine treatment, should be considered in addition to the intensive physical health monitoring recommended in adults.
- The risks and benefits of clozapine should be fully discussed with the child, parents or guardians and this should be followed up by appropriate written information.

Further reading and resources

Findling R, Frazier J, Gerbino-Rosen G, Kranzler H, Kumra S, Kratochvil C. Is there a role for clozapine in the treatment of children and adolescents? *J Am Acad Child Adolesc Psychiatry* 2007; **46:** 423–8

For patient and carer friendly advice on psychotropics including clozapine visit: www.choiceandmedication.org

References

1. Findling R, Frazier J, Gerbino-Rosen G, Kranzler H, Kumra S, Kratochvil C. Is there a role for clozapine in the treatment of children and adolescents? *J Am Acad Child Adolesc Psychiatry* 2007; **46:** 423–8
2. Gogtay N, Rapoport J. Clozapine use in children and adolescents. *Expert Opin Pharmacother* 2008; **9:** 459–65
3. Masi G, Mucci M, Pari C. Children with schizophrenia. Clinical picture and pharmacological treatment. *CNS Drugs* 2006; **20:** 841–66
4. Kumra S, Oberstar J, Sikich L, Findling R, McClellan J, Vinogradov S, et al. Efficacy and tolerability of second-generation antipsychotics in children and adolescents with schizophrenia. *Schizophr Bull* 2008; **34:** 60–71
5. Kumra S, Kranzler H, Gerbino-Rosen G, Kester HM, Dethomas C, Kafantaris V, et al. Clozapine and 'high-dose' olanzapine in refractory early-onset schizophrenia: A 12-week randomized and double-blind comparison. *Biol Psychiatry* 2008; **63:** 524–9
6. Shaw P, Sporn A, Gotay N, Overman G, Greenstein D, Gochman P, et al. Childhood-onset schizophrenia. A double-blind, randonized clozapine-olanzapine comparison. *Arch Gen Psychiatry* 2006; **63:** 721–30
7. Kumra S, Frazier J, Jacobsen L, McKenna K, Gordon C, Lenane M, et al. Childhood-onset schizophrenia. A double-blind clozapine-haloperidol comparison. *Arch Gen Psychiatry* 1996; **53:** 1090–7
8. National Institute for Health and Clinical Excellence. *Psychosis and schizophrenia in children and young people.* CG155 January 2013 . Available at: http://www.nice.org.uk
9. Kumra S, Kranzler H, Gerbino-Rosen G, Kester H, DeThomas C, Cullen K, et al. Clozapine versus 'high-dose' olanzapine in refractory early-onset schizophrenia: An open-label extension study. *J Child Adolesc Psychopharmacol* 2008; **18:** 307–16
10. Kim Y, Kim BN, Cho SC, Kim JW, Shin MS. Long-term sustained benefits of clozapine treatment in refractory early onset schizophrenia: A retrospective study in Korean children and adolescents. *Hum Psychopharmacol* 2008; **23:** 715–22
11. Sporn A, Vermani A, Greenstein D, Bobb A, Spencer E, Clasen L, et al. Clozapine treatment of childhood-onset schizophrenia: Evaluation of effectiveness, adverse effects and long-term outcome. *J Am Acad Child Adolesc Psychiatry* 2007; **46:** 1349–56
12. Kranzler H, Roofeh D, Gerbino-Rosen G, Dombrowski C, McMeneman M, DeThomas C, et al. Clozapine: Its impact on aggressive behaviour among children and adolescents with schizophrenia. *J Am Acad Child Adolesc Psychiatry* 2005; **44:** 55–63
13. Turetz M, Mozes T, Toren P, Chernauzan N, Yoran-Hegesh R, Mester R, et al. An Open trial of clozapine in neuroleptic-resistant childhood-onset schizophrenia. *Br J Psychiatry* 1997; **170:** 507–10

14. Frazer J, Gordon C, McKenna K, Lenane M, Jih D, Rapoport J. An open trial of clozapine in 11 adolescents with childhood-onset schizophrenia. *J Am Acad Child Adolesc Psychiatry* 1994; **33:** 658–63
15. Masi G, Mucci M, Millepiedi S. Clozapine in adolescent inpatients with acute mania. *J Am Acad Child Adolesc Psychiatry* 2002; **12:** 93–9
16. Beherec L, Lambrey S, Quilici G, Rosier A, Falissard B, Guilin O. Retrospective review of clozapine in the treatment of patients with autism spectrum disorders and severe disruptive behaviours. *J Clin Psychopharmacol* 2011; **31:** 341–4
17. Teixeria E, Santos A, Salán T, Jacintho A, Celeri E, Dalgalarrondo P. The use of clozapine in children and adolescents with serious conduct disorder for control of the aggressiveness. *Eur Psychiatry* 2010; **25(suppl 1):** 995
18. Correll C, Carlson H. Endocrine and metabolic adverse effects of psychotropic medications in children and adolescents. *J Am Acad Child Adolesc Psychiatry* 2006; **45:** 771–91
19. Sporn A, Bobb A, Gogtay N, Stevens H, Greenstein D, Clasen L, et al. Hormonal correlates of clozapine-induced weight gain in psychotic children: An exploratory study. *J Am Acad Child Adolesc Psychiatry* 2005; **44:** 925–33
20. David C, Maher K, Tan M, Tossell J, Weisinger B, Gochman P, et al. Risk factors for neutropenia in clozapine-treated children and adolescents with childhood-onset schizophrenia. *Biol Psychiatry* 2012; **71(suppl 1):** 102S
21. Couchman L, Bowskill S, Handley S, Patel M, Flanagan R. Plasma clozapine and norclozapine in relation to prescribed dose and other factors in patients aged <18 years: data from a therapeutic drug monitoring service, 1994–2010. *Early Interv Psychiatry* 2012; **7:** 122–30
22. Clozaril specific product characteristics (SPC). Novartis. Available at: www.medicines.org.uk (accessed December 2012)
23. Royal College of Psychiatrists. Use of unlicenced medicines for unlicensed applications in psychiatry. College Report CR142. January 2007
24. Cirulli G. Clozapine prescribing in adolescent psychiatry: survey of prescribing practice in in-patient units. *Psychiatr Bull* 2005; **29:** 377–80

10.7: Seizures and EEG changes

Clozapine is a well-known pro-convulsant agent which appears to present a higher risk of inducing seizures than other antipsychotics[1,2]. According to the World Health Organization's (WHO) adverse drug reaction database, clozapine is in the top five of neuroactive agents associated with seizures[3].

Clozapine and seizures

Clozapine-induced seizures are both dose-related and related to the speed of titration. In an early study by Devinsky et al, 41 of 1,418 (2.9%) patients had a generalised tonic-clonic seizure. High dose therapy (>=600mg/day) was associated with a greater risk of seizures (4.4%) than medium doses (300-600mg/day, 2.7% risk) or low doses (<300mg/day, 1% risk)[4]. Thirty-one of the 41 patients were successfully continued on clozapine despite seizures. All 31 had their dose reduced and 15 of the 31 had an antiepileptic medication co-prescribed. Devinsky et al predicted a cumulative 10% risk of seizures after a mean of 3.8 years of clozapine treatment[4]. Other studies have reported a seizure rate as low as 1%[5] or as high as 10%[6] in inpatients. Having a previous history of seizures[5,6] or head trauma[5] may increase the risk of clozapine-induced seizures. In the largest investigation to date (n=5,629), a dose-dependent risk for seizures was not demonstrated. However, this may be partially explained by a high number of patients with a history of seizures in the low dose group (<300mg/day)[6]. Although tonic-clonic seizures are the seizure type most often reported with clozapine, myoclonic jerks, atonic seizures, drop attacks and even stuttering[7,8] have been reported and may be a precursor to tonic-clonic seizures[9].

The mechanism by which clozapine lowers the seizure threshold is not fully understood. Clozapine commonly causes electroencephalographic (EEG) changes which are usually non-specific and not indicative of seizures (see below)[10]. It is unlikely to be due to dopamine antagonism because clozapine is thought to have a

Figure 10.7.1: Risk factors associated with clozapine related seizures[3,4,5,6]

Clozapine factors	Comorbid factors
Clozapine dose (≥600mg/day or level≥500mcgs/L), but note seizures can occur at any dose or level Rapid dose escalation Deliberate or unintentional overdose	History of seizures History of head trauma Concurrent epileptogenic medication (e.g. chlorpromazine, clomipramine etc) Stopping smoking (and the resulting elevation in clozapine levels) Concurrent enzymes inhibitors (which increase clozapine levels) General physical illness (e.g. hypoglycaemia, hyponatreamia, infection, hypertensive encephalopathy, etc) Alcohol or drug misuse

higher affinity for blocking D_1 receptors (which may protect against seizures) than D_2 receptors (which are associated with seizures)[3, 11]. *In vitro* experiments have suggested that clozapine acts as a $GABA_A$ (gamma-aminobutyric acid) antagonist in the ventral tegmental area, and this mechanism may be implicated in seizures[12]. Another hypothesis links the increase in leptin seen with clozapine as a potential cause of increased seizures[13]. All we can really say is that clozapine appears to be associated with seizures more than other antipsychotics and this probably reflects its broad and unique receptor profile.

Clozapine and EEG changes

Although clozapine commonly causes abnormal changes in EEGs, the clinical significance of this is uncertain. As many as 50–60% of those exposed to clozapine show abnormalities which are most often reported as non-specific slow waves[10, 14]. Relatively few patients however, go on to develop seizures. The EEG slowing generally occurs more frequently and more severely with an increased clozapine dose and may be related to sedation[10, 14]. Varma et al in 2011 conducted a regression analysis of studies reporting on EEG changes with clozapine. They concluded that each 100mg increase in clozapine dose was associated with an 8% increase in the number of patients with an abnormal EEG (p=0.022)[15]. Clozapine plasma levels were also investigated and the authors discovered that each 100mcg/L increase in clozapine level was associated with a 12% increase in the number of patients with an abnormal EEG (p=0.023)[15].

Some authors have proposed that an abnormal EEG with clozapine is a marker of better clinical response[16]. However, this has not been studied in any depth.

Routine EEG monitoring with clozapine is probably not warranted in the general population, but may be useful in those who have a higher risk for seizures (e.g. those with a history of epilepsy, head trauma and for children and adolescents). Any EEG taken should be thoroughly reviewed for epiletiform activity by an appropriately experienced clinician.

Treatment of clozapine-induced seizures

If a patient has a seizure while receiving clozapine, it is usually recommended to withhold the dose for 24 hours then reintroduce at a lower dose[17] (a 50% dose reduction has been suggested by the manufacturers). An EEG and referral to a neurologist might be considered, especially if this is the patient's first seizure. Dose reduction may be sufficient to prevent another seizure, but for those who will need to be re-titrated to a higher dose or who have recurrent seizures, an anticonvulsant should be used. Many anticonvulsants have been used for clozapine-induced seizures (*Table 10.7.1*). Valproate is the most commonly used and widely accepted[15], but remains underutilised in those at risk[18].

Table 10.7.1: Anticonvulsants used in clozapine-related seizures

Author	Anticonvulsant/ dose at maintance	Number of patients	Comment
Foster et al, 2005[19]	Sodium valproate 500mg/day	1	Widely regarded as the drug of choice for clozapine-induced seizures. Broad spectrum of anticonvulsant activity. Mood stabiliser and anti-manic properties[15]
Meltzer et al, 1994[20]	Valproic acid 1500mg/ day	1	Valproate is an established human teratogen[22] and therefore should be avoided in women of child-bearing age. If valproate cannot be avoided, appropriate contraception should be recommended and prophylactic folic acid prescribed. First trimester exposure, higher doses and polytherapy constitute the greatest risks[23]
Tanner el al, 1998[21]	Valproic acid 800mg/day (case 1), 1000mg/day (case 2)	2	Valproate may increase or decrease clozapine/norclozapine plasma levels, but the effects appear to be modest at most and largely insignificant[24]
Muzki et al, 2010[25]	Lamotrigine 200mg / day	1	Slow onset of action due to initial gradual titration. A rash generally in the first 8 weeks of treatment is common, although usually mild. However, life-threatening rashes such as Stevens-Johnston syndrome and toxic epidermal necrosis have been reported[26] A useful augmentation strategy in treatment–resistant schizophrenia for inadequate responders to clozapine alone[27]. Has mood stabilising and antidepressant properties[15] Unlikely to cause pharmacokinetic drug interactions with clozapine
Navarro et al, 2001[28]	Topiramate 200mg/day	1	Requires a gradual dose titration to test for tolerability. Common adverse reactions include cognitive dysfunction, mood changes and visual disturbances[29] Can induce weight loss Unlikely to cause pharmacokinetic drug interactions with clozapine
Usiskin et al, 2000[30]	Gabapentin 2100mg/day	1	May be an option if other anticonvulsants poorly tolerated. Dosing adjustments are recommended in those with renal impairment[32]
Landry et al, 2001[31]	Gabapentin 1200mg / day	1	May have anxiolytic properties[15] Unlikely to cause pharmacokinetic drug interactions with clozapine

Valproate has well recognised mood stabiliser and anti-manic properties, but should be avoided in women of child-bearing potential because of the link with neonatal malformations. Lamotrigine is a suitable alternative and may be particularly useful in those only partly responsive to clozapine (it is often used as an augmenting agent). Those prescribed lamotrigine for the first time should be closely monitored for a rash which, although usually mild, can rarely rapidly worsen. In other respects, lamotrigine is usually well tolerated. Gabapentin and topiramate are possible choices where valproate or lamotrigine are not appropriate. Other anticonvulsants used in clozapine-induced seizures include phenytoin, phenobarbitone and carbamazepine[4, 5]. All three are hepatically metabolised and potent inducers of the cytochrome P450 isoenzymes CYP1A2 and CYP3A4. This would be expected to reduce clozapine plasma levels and require the clozapine dose to be increased to maintain efficacy[24]. Carbamazepine (and to a lesser extent phenytoin and phenobarbitone), are associated with bone marrow suppression, including agranulocytosis, and would pose a significant risk if used in conjunction with clozapine.

Preventing clozapine-induced seizures

Although the risk of seizures generally rises with increasing clozapine dose and plasma level, seizures can occur at any time during treatment. For those with prominent risk factors (*Figure 10.7.1*), clear epiletiform discharges on the EEG, or if the patient develops stuttering or myloclonic jerks, prophylaxic anticonvulsants should be considered. Using the lowest effective clozapine dose, ensuring a gradual initial titration and avoiding concurrent epileptogenic medicines will also reduce the risk of seizures[15].

Clozapine use in epilepsy

For those with a diagnosis of epilepsy and treatment resistant-psychosis, clozapine is a viable option with close monitoring for increased frequency and duration of seizures. Before initiating clozapine, the anticonvulsant should be reviewed to ensure good seizure control and to minimise potential interactions[33]. Clozapine should be initiated slowly and the lowest effective dose used to reduce the risk of destabilising seizures. Monitoring clozapine plasma levels and EEGs is recommended to guide dosing and monitor tolerability. A collaborative approach between neurology and psychiatry services will also help ensure consistency in treatment. Although epilepsy might be a formal contraindication to clozapine use, there have been many successful uses of clozapine in people with a variety of pre-existing seizure disorders[35].

Clozapine and electroconvulsive therapy (ECT)

The final issue to consider in this section is the contentious use of clozapine alongside electroconvulsive therapy (ECT). ECT is occasionally used in schizophrenia for rapid symptom relief or where antipsychotics alone have shown a limited response[34, 36]. Clozapine, along with all epileptogenic medication, has the potential to prolong seizures during and after ECT sessions. Data relating to combined ECT and clozapine therapy are scarce, largely limited to case reports or case series. In the largest studies, the combination is generally well tolerated and effective. Kupchik et al[37] reported on 36 patients treated with both ECT and clozapine. The mean dose of clozapine was 385mg/day (±172mg), while the number of ECT sessions was 12 (±6). They concluded that the combined treatment was more effective than either treatment alone and 67.2% of patients showed an improvement. Adverse reactions occurred in 16.6% of patients and these included one case of a prolonged seizure and one case of supraventricular and sinus tachycardia[37]. In a preliminary report of the first RCT comparing clozapine alone with clozapine and ECT, 10 of 21 (48%) in the combined arm demonstrated a response. The author reported the combination was generally well tolerated with no unusual adverse events observed[38]. There is also a case series (n=28) supporting the combined use of clozapine and ECT in adolescents (between 13–18-year-olds) with schizophrenia spectrum disorder[39].

When considering the combined use of clozapine and ECT, clinicians should be mindful of the many physical health effects associated with clozapine which can complicate the ECT procedure.

Summary

- Clozapine commonly causes abnormal EEG changes but relatively few patients (between 1–10%) will develop seizures.
- Seizures can occur at any time while prescribed clozapine. The risk is highest during the initial stages of titration and at high doses.
- Interacting drugs or substances which increase clozapine levels can also heighten the risk of a seizure.
- Following a seizure, clozapine should be stopped for 24 hours and re-introduced at a lower dose, and slowly titrated to clinical effect (plasma level monitoring is essential).
- For those with recurrent seizures or at a considerable risk of a seizure, an anticonvulsant such as lamotrigine or valproate should be considered.
- Lamotrigine is often preferred to valproate, but must be used cautiously because of the association with a severe rash.

Further reading

Varma S, Bishara D, Besag F, Taylor D. Clozapine-related EEG changes and seizures: dose and plasma-level relationships. *Ther Adv Psychopharmacol* 2011; **1**: 47–66

References

1. Murphy K, Delanty N. Drug-induced seizures. General principles in assessment, management and prevention. *CNS Drugs* 2000; **14:** 135–46

2. Pisani F, Oteri G, Costa C, Di Raimondo G, Di Perri R. Effects of psychotropic drugs on seizure threshold. *Drug Safety* 2002; **25:** 91–110

3. Kumlien E, Lundberg P. Seizure risk associated with neuroactive drugs: data from the WHO adverse drug reaction database. *Seizure* 2010; **19:** 69–73

4. Devinsky O, Honigfeld G, Patin J. Clozapine-related seizures. *Neurology* 1991; **41:** 369–71

5. Wilson W, Claussen A. Seizures associated with clozapine treatment in a state hospital. *J Clin Psychiatry* 1994; **55:** 184–8

6. Pacia S, Devinsky O. Clozapine-related seizures. Experience with 5,629 patients. *Neurology* 1994; **44:** 2247–9

7. Supprian T, Retz W, Deckert J. Clozapine-induced stuttering: Epileptic brain activity? *Am J Psychiatry* 1999; **156:** 1663

8. Begum M. Clozapine-induced stuttering, facial tics and myoclonic seizures: A case report. *Aust N Z J Psychiatry* 2005; **39:** 202

9. Wong J, Delva N. Clozapine-induced seizures: Recognition and treatment. *Can J Psychiatry* 2007; **52:** 457–63

10. Chung SJ, Jeong SH, Ahn YM, Kang UG, Koo YJ, Ha JH, et al. A retrospective study of clozapine and electroencephalographic abnormalities in schizophrenic patients. *Prog Neurologypsychopharmacol Biol Psychiatry* 2002; **26:** 139–44

11. Meltzer HY. Clinical studies on the mechanism of action of clozapine: the dopamine-serotonin hypothesis of schizophrenia. *Psychopharmacology* (Berl) 1989; **99(Suppl):** S18–S27

12. Michel F, Trudeau L. Clozapine inhibits synaptic transmission at GABAergic synapses established by ventral tegmental area neurones in culture. *Neuropharmacology* 2000; **39:** 1536–43

13. Ghanizadeh A. Modulation of leptin by histamine H1 receptors as a novel therapeutic approach for treatment of clozapine induced seizures. *Psychiatr Danubina* 2010; **22:** 552–3

14. Freudenreich O, weiner R, McEvoy J. Clozapine-induced electroencephalogram changes as a function of clozapine serum levels. *Biol Psychiatry* 1997; **42:** 132–7

15. Varma S, Bishara D, Besag F, Taylor D. Clozapine-related EEG changes and seizures: dose and plasma-level relationships. *Ther Adv Psychopharmacol* 2011; **1:** 47–66

16. Koukkou M, Angst J, Zimmer D. Paroxysmal EEG activity and psychopathology during treatment with clozapine. *Pharmacopsychiatry* 1979; **12:** 173–83

17. Taylor D, Paton C, Kapur S. *The Maudsley Prescribing guidelines* 11th edn: Chichester: Wiley-Blackwell: 2012

18. Sparshatt A, Whiskey E, Taylor D. Valproate as prophylaxis for clozapine-induced seizures: survey of practice. *Psychiatr Bull* 2008; **32:** 262–5

19. Foster R, Olajide D. A case of clozapine-induced tonic-clonic seizures managed with valproate: implications for clinical care. *J Psychopharmacol* 2005; **19:** 83–96

20. Meltzer H, Ranjan R. Valproic acid treatment of clozapine-induced myoclonus. *Am J Psychiatry* 1994; **151:** 1246–7

21. Tanner E, Cosar B, Isik E. Clozapine-induced myoclonic seizures and valproic acid. *Int J Psychiatry Clin Practice* 1998; **2:** 53–5
22. Wyszynski D, Nambisan M, Surve T, Alsdorf R, Smith C, Holmes L, et al. Increased rate of major malformations in offspring exposed to valproate during pregnancy. *Neurology* 2005; **64:** 938–9
23. National Institute for Health and Clinical Excellence. *The epilepsies: the diagnosis and management of the epilepsies in adult and children in primary and secondary care, Clinical Guideline 137.* Available at: http://www.nice.org.uk. 2012 (accessed December 2012)
24. Baxter K. *Stockley's Drug Interactions* 9th edn. London : Pharmaceutical Press: 2010
25. Muzyk A, Gala G, Khan D. Use of lamotrigine in a patient with a clozapine-related seizure. *J Psychiatr Practice* 2010; **16:** 125–8
26. Lamictal specific product characteristics (SPC). GlaxoSmithKline UK. Available at: www.medicines.org.uk (accessed 21 December 2012)
27. Tiihonen J, Wahlbeck K, Kiviniemi V. The efficacy of lamotrigine in clozapine-resistant schizophrenia: A systematic review and meta-analysis. *Schizophr Res* 2009; **109:** 10–14
28. Navarro V, Pons A, Romero A, Bernardo M. Topiramate for clozapine-induced seizures. *Am J Psychiatry* 2001; **158:** 968–9
29. Topamax specific product characteristics (SPC). Janssen-Cilag Ltd. Available at: www.medicines.org.uk (accessed 21 December 2012)
30. Usiskin S, Nicolson R, Lenane M, Rapoport J. Gabapentin prophylaxis of clozapine-induced seizures. *Am J Psychiatry* 2000; **157:** 482–3
31. Landry P. Gabapentin for clozapine-related seizures. *Am J Psychiatry* 2001; **158:** 1930–1
32. Gabapentin specific product characteristics (SPC). Sandoz Ltd. Available at: www.medicines.org.uk (accessed 21 December 2012)
33. Langosch J, Trimble M. Epilepsy, psychosis and clozapine. *Hum Psychopharmacol* 2002; **17:** 115–19
34. Tharyan P, Adams CE. Electroconvulsive therapy for schizophrenia. Cochrane Database of Systematic Reviews 2005, Issue 2. Art. No.: CD000076. DOI: 10.1002/14651858.CD000076.pub2
35. Langosch J, Trimble M. Epilepsy, psychosis and clozapine. *Hum Psychopharmacol Clin Experimental* 2002; **17:** 115–9
36. Royal College of Psychiatrists Special Committee on ECT. *The ECT handbook* 2nd edn, CR128; London: The Royal College of Psychiatrists: 2005
37. Kupchik M, Spivak B, Mester R, Reznik I, Gonen N, Weizman A, et al. Combined electroconvulsive-clozapine therapy. *Clin Neuropharmacol* 2000; **23:** 14–16
38. Braga R, Mendelowitz A, Fink M, Schooler N, Bailine S, Malur C, et al. A randomized controlled trial of ECT in clozapine-refractory schizophrenia. *Biol Psychiatry* 2009; **64:** 1S–244S
39. Itziar F, Josefina CF, Miguel G, Elena d, Alexandre P, Miguel B, et al. Electroconvulsive therapy and clozapine in adolescents with schizophrenia spectrum disorder: Is it a safe and effective combination? *J Clin Psychopharmacol* 2012; **32:** 756–66

11. Post-mortem

A great many drugs are subject to post-mortem effects but, for obvious practical reasons, research into the mechanisms and extent of these effects is limited. The best that can be said is that a drug plasma level during life is often different from the (usually whole blood) concentration measured some time after death.

A number of processes are responsible for these changes in concentration. In life, active mechanisms serve to concentrate some drugs in certain organs or tissues. After death, passive diffusion occurs and this often means that central blood vessels show much higher concentrations than peripheral samples. This and other processes are time-dependent, and so time since death is an important determinant of blood concentration changes. The effect of redistribution tends to be greater with drugs with a large volume of distribution (i.e. those for which tissue concentrations in life vastly exceed blood concentrations)[1].

Other processes of importance include synthesis of certain compounds (the body can generate gamma-hydroxy butyrate and bacteria involved in putrefaction can produce alcohol) and degradation by bacteria (clonazepam and nitrazepam are transformed by bacteria). The metabolism of some drugs (cocaine, for example) continues after death.

Clozapine has a large volume of distribution (often cited as being greater than 5L/kg), which implies that most of the body's stores of clozapine are outside the blood compartment. As such, clozapine would be expected to show both a wide peripheral/central blood compartment differential post-mortem and to exhibit post-mortem redistribution (from tissues and organs into the blood compartment).

Evidence regarding clozapine's fate after death began to emerge only in the 1990s. An early case series[2] described hepatic concentrations of clozapine to be roughly 10–30 times higher than femoral blood or muscle concentrations. At around the same time, a death due to clozapine overdose was reported[3]. In this case, twenty 100mg tablets were ingested and a resultant plasma level of 1,940ng/ml measured four hours later. The subject died two hours after this and analysis of heart blood found a (eight hours) post-mortem concentration of 5,810ng/ml — almost three times the concentration measured while still alive. This increase could not be explained by absorption from ingested clozapine between plasma sampling and death because gastric lavage was carried out at the same time as sampling. A further case reported in 2004[4] showed a similar change: in life concentrations averaged around 600ng/ml, but a central post-mortem sample showed a concentration of 1700ng/ml. These observations were further supported by an analysis of 21 cases where both ante-mortem and post-mortem clozapine concentrations had been measured[5] — mean in-life concentration was 600ng/ml; mean post-mortem level 2,760ng/ml (a factor of 4.6). Before and after concentrations were strongly related (R^2=0.31).

The largest increase in clozapine concentration reported was from a case of death occurring as a result of gastrointestinal hypomotility[6]. The patient had a serum concentration of 560ng/ml during life and a level of 3,730ng/ml in femoral whole blood <34 hours post-mortem (i.e. increased by a factor of 6.66).

There is only one prospective study of clozapine concentrations before and after death and this was in pigs (as a model for human effects)[7]. Two pigs were given clozapine for a week and then sacrificed. Plasma (ante-mortem) and whole blood (post-mortem) concentrations were determined for both animals. Post-mortem sampling continued for 48 hours after death. Overall, measured concentrations of clozapine increased as a function of time since death. In central blood, concentrations were increased by a factor of around 2 at four hours, and by a factor of around 3 at 48 hours. For peripheral samples, there was a less clear relationship between concentration and time of sampling and concentrations reached only 1.5 times their in-life values. The study also showed a massive time-dependent increase in organ concentrations of clozapine post-mortem. A separate experiment described in the paper compared concentration of clozapine in whole blood and plasma in a single human volunteer. Concentrations were slightly higher (~10%) in plasma than in whole blood. This suggests that increased concentrations found in whole blood post-mortem reflect a somewhat greater degree of re-distribution than if plasma and blood concentrations were equal.

These observed changes in clozapine concentrations are of considerable importance in determining cause of death in patients receiving clozapine. Coroners may erroneously implicate clozapine as the sole or major cause of death when post-mortem concentrations are found to be in the toxic range (perhaps >1000ng/ml)[8]. As we have seen, because of redistribution, central blood post-mortem concentrations are likely to appear 'toxic' in any patient with a therapeutic plasma concentration (>350ng/ml) in life. Any interpretation of post-mortem concentrations should consider post-mortem distribution and the effects of time[9], temperature of body storage, site of sampling and other factors on the extent of redistribution[10].

Summary

- Clozapine is a drug with a large volume of distribution and this predicts changes in tissue and blood concentrations after death.
- In post-mortem whole blood, clozapine concentrations may be increased by a factor of 1.5 (peripheral blood) or around 3–7 (central blood).
- Post-mortem concentrations increase as a function of time since death.
- Post-mortem clozapine concentrations need to be carefully interpreted to avoid falsely implicating clozapine poisoning as the cause of death.

References

1. Kennedy MC. Post-mortem drug concentrations. *Intern Med J* 2010; **40:**183–7
2. Worm K, Kringsholm B, Steentoft A. Clozapine cases with fatal, toxic or therapeutic concentrations. *Int J Legal Med* 1993; **106:**115–18
3. Meeker JE, Herrmann PW, Som CW, Reynolds PC. Clozapine tissue concentrations following an apparent suicidal overdose of Clozaril. *J Anal Toxicol* 1992; **16:** 54–6
4. de Leon J, Simpson GM. Postmortem clozapine levels. *J Clin Psychopharmacol* 2004; **24:** 100–1
5. Flanagan RJ, Spencer EP, Morgan PE, Barnes TR, Dunk L. Suspected clozapine poisoning in the UK/Eire, 1992–2003. *Forensic Sci Int* 2005; **155:** 91–9
6. Flanagan RJ, Ball RY. Gastrointestinal hypomotility: an under-recognised life-threatening adverse effect of clozapine. *Forensic Sci Int* 2011; **206:** e31–e36
7. Flanagan RJ, Amin A, Seinen W. Effect of post-mortem changes on peripheral and central whole blood and tissue clozapine and norclozapine concentrations in the domestic pig (Sus scrofa). *Forensic Sci Int* 2003; **132:** 9–17
8. Jaskiw GE, Konicki PE, Fuller MA. Clozapine: toxicity vs. postmortem redistribution. *Schizophr Res* 2008; **101:** 344–5
9. Saar E, Beyer J, Gerostamoulos D, Drummer OH. The time-dependant post-mortem redistribution of antipsychotic drugs. *Forensic Sci Int* 2012; **222:** 223–7
10. Stark A, Scott J. A review of the use of clozapine levels to guide treatment and determine cause of death. *Aust N Z J Psychiatry* 2012; **46:** 816–25

Appendix 1.

Worldwide availability

The availability of medicines across the World changes rapidly. National regulation and advice is also subject to sudden change. Therefore, the following table should be regarded for interest only and readers are strongly recommended to check on the current situation.

In general, the UK, US, Canada, Australia, New Zealand, and Ireland have a similar monitoring system where the prescriber, pharmacy and patient are registered with the company and the company and pharmacy closely monitor blood test results before dispensing (the frequency of monitoring differs). There is also some consistency in the wording and content of clozapine product literature across the European Union, although again the frequency and who conducts the monitoring is subject to change[1].

Table Appendix 1.1[1,2,3]

Country	Clozapine availability	Brands available	Company (monitoring service website)	WBC monitoring frequency
Australia	Widely available	Clozaril®	Clozaril® Novartis Pharmaceuticals Australia www.novartis.com.au	Weekly for the first 18 weeks, 4-weekly thereafter.
		Clopine®	Clopine® Mayne Pharma Pty Ltd Company website: http://www.clopine.com.au For the consumer medicines information leaflet (CMI) visit: www.medicines.org.au	Company monitoring system
Canada	Widely available	Clozaril®	Clozaril® Novartis Pharmaceuticals Canada Inc. www.csan.ca	Weekly for 26 weeks, then 2-weekly for 26 weeks, and 4-weekly thereafter
		Apo-Clozapine®	Apo-clozapine® Apotex Inc www.apoclozapine.com	Company monitoring system
		Gen-Clozapine®	Gen-Clozapine® Mylan www.gencan.ca	
Denmark	Widely available	Leponex® Many generic preparations available	Leponex® Novartis Denmark www.novartis.dk	Weekly for 18 weeks, then 4-weekly

Country	Clozapine availability	Brands available	Company (monitoring service website)	WBC monitoring frequency
Denmark, *continued*	Widely available	Leponex® Many generic preparations available	Leponex® Novartis Denmark www.novartis.dk	No formal company monitoring or pharmacy regulation. Prescribers are expected to ensure full blood counts are competed before prescribing. Any Doctor can prescribe clozapine and any pharmacy is able to supply
Finland	Widely available	Leponex® Many generic preparations available	Leponex® Novartis Finland www.novartis.fi	Weekly for 18 weeks, then 4-weekly No formal company monitoring or pharmacy regulation. Prescribers are expected to ensure full blood counts are competed before prescribing. Any doctor can prescribe clozapine and any pharmacy is able to supply
France	Widely available	Leponex® Generic preparations available	Leponex® Novartis Pharma SAS www.novartis.fr Generic clozapine Panpharma www.panpharma.fr	Weekly for the first 18 weeks, 4-weekly thereafter No formal company monitoring service, but blood monitoring is checked by the supplying pharmacy before dispensing Initiation is generally in hospital only by a psychiatrist, neurologist or geriatrician. Any pharmacy can supply following a valid blood test
Germany	Widely available	Leponex® Generic preparations available	Leponex® Deutchland www.novartis.de	Weekly for the first 18 weeks, 4-weekly thereafter Any doctor is able to prescribe and any pharmacy can supply clozapine
India	Widely available	Many generic preparations available		Treating physician dictates the monitoring. No National monitoring service. Any pharmacy is able to stock clozapine

Country	Clozapine availability	Brands available	Company (monitoring service website)	WBC monitoring frequency
Ireland	Widely available	Clozaril®	Clozaril® Novartis Ireland www.clozaril.co.uk	Weekly for the first 18 weeks, 2-weekly weeks 18–52, 4-weekly thereafter
		Denzapine® Denzapine® oral solution 50mg/ml	Denzapine® Merz Pharma UK Ltd www.denzapine.co.uk The specific product characteristics are available at: www.medicines.ie	Company monitoring system
Italy	Widely available	Leponex® Generic preparations available	Leponex® Novartis Italy	Weekly for the first 18 weeks, then 4-weekly
			Clozapina: Hexal SPA Clozapina: Chiesi Farmaceutici SPA The specific product characteristics are available at: www.doctoralia.it	No formal monitoring system
New Zealand	Widely available	Clozaril®	Clozaril® Carelink Novartis New Zealand Ltd	Weekly for the first 18 weeks, 4-weekly thereafter
		Clopine® Clopine® oral suspension 50mg/ml	Clopine® Douglas Pharmaceuticals Ltd For the consumer medicines information leaflet (CMI) visit: http://www.medsafe.govt.nz	The supplying pharmacy monitors WBC counts
Spain	Widely available	Leponex®	Leponex® Novartis Spain www.novartis.es	Weekly for the first 18 weeks, then 4-weekly. Psychiatrists only are able to prescribe, but any pharmacy can supply The health authority controls blood test monitoring
UK	Widely available	Clozaril®	Clozaril® - Novartis Pharmaceuticals UK Ltd www.clozaril.co.uk	Weekly for the first 18 weeks, 2-weekly weeks 18–52, 4-weekly thereafter

Country	Clozapine availability	Brands available	Company (monitoring service website)	WBC monitoring frequency
UK	Widely available	Denzapine® Denzapine® oral solution 50mg/ml Zaponex ®	Denzapine® Genus Pharmaceuticals www.denzapine.co.uk Zaponex® Layden Delta BV http://www.ztas.co.uk The specific product characteristics are available at: www.medicines.org.uk	Company monitoring system
US	Widely available	Clozaril® FazClo® oral disintegrating tablets Many generic preparations available	Clozaril® Novartis Pharmaceuticals Corporation www.clozaril.com FazClo® Azur Pharma Inc www.fazclo.com Generic clozapine, Mylan www.mylan-clozapine.com Generic clozapine, Teva www.clozapineregistry.com For the package insert visit: fbd.rxlist.com/drug	Weekly for first 6 months, then 2-weekly for 6 months, and 4-weekly thereafter Company monitoring system
Novartis are a global company with a presence in over 40 countries. If the country you are looking for is not listed above, the authors recommend that you contact Novartis directly (www.novartis.com)				

References

1. The European agency for the evaluation of medicinal products. Committee for proprietary medicinal products. Summary information on referral opinion following arbitration. Leponex and associated names. London 12 November 2002 (available at www.ema.europa.eu/)
2. Clozaril Patient Monitoring Service (CPMS). Personal communication 27 December 2012
3. Martindale: *The Complete Drug Reference*. [online] London: Pharmaceutical Press. www.medicinescomplete.com (accessed on 27 December 2012)

Appendix 2.

Signposting and useful links

National mental health charities/organisations

UK

www.sane.org.uk	A National mental health charity
www.rethink.org	A National charity for anyone affected by mental illness
www.mind.org.uk	A National charity for anyone affected by mental illness

Ireland

www.mentalhealthireland.ie	A National voluntary organisation
www.headstrong.ie	The National Centre for youth Mental Health

Australia

www.sane.org	A National charity supporting all affected by mental illness
www.sfnsw.org.au	The Schizophrenia Fellowship

New Zealand

www.mentalhealth.org.nz	Mental Health Foundation of New Zealand
www.supportingfamilies.org.nz	Supporting families in mental illness.

US

www.mentalhealthamerica.net	Mental Health America
www.nami.org	The National Alliance on Mental Illness
bbrfoundation.org	The Brain and Behaviour research foundation

Canada

www.cmha.ca	The Canadian Mental Health Association
www.schizophrenia.ca	Schizophrenia Society of Canada

Others

www.mhe-sme.org	Mental Health Europe
www.wfmh.org	World Federation for Mental Health

National medicines regulatory authorities

UK

www.mhra.gov.uk	The Medicines and Healthcare Products Regulatory Authority

Europe wide

www.ema.europa.eu	The European Medicines Agency

US

www.fda.gov	The US Food and Drug Administration

Australia

www.tga.gov.au	The Therapeutic Goods Association

New Zealand

http://www.medsafe.govt.nz	New Zealand Medicines and Medical Devices Safety Authority.

Canada

www.hc-sc.gc.ca	Health Canada

Ireland

www.imb.ie	The Irish Medicines Board

France

ansm.sante.fr	The French National Agency of Medicines and Health Products Safety

Germany

www.bfarm.de	The Federal Institute for Drugs and Medical Devices

National professional bodies in psychiatry

UK

www.rcpsych.org.uk	The Royal College of Psychiatrists UK
www.bap.org.uk	The British Association for Psychopharmacology
www.cmhp.org.uk	The College of Mental Health Pharmacy

Ireland

www.irishpsychiatry.ie	The College of Psychiatry Ireland

Australia and New Zealand

www.ranzcp.org	The Royal Australian and New Zealand College of Psychiatrists

US

www.psychiatry.org	The American Psychiatric Association
cpnp.org	The College of Psychiatric and Neurologic Pharmacists

Canada

www.cpa-apc.org	Canadian Psychiatric Association

others

www.ecnp.eu	European College of Neuropsychopharmacology

Patient/carer information

www.choiceandmedication.org.uk	Reliable and impartial information on all medicines for mental illness.
www.nhsdirect.nhs.uk	Accessible healthcare information
www.patient.co.uk	Patient information/publications

National guidelines in mental health

www.nice.org.uk	The National Institute for Health and Clinical Excellence (available as an app)
www.sign.ac.uk	The Scottish Intercollegiate Guidelines Network
http://www.guidelines.gov	US Department of Health and Human Services (National Guideline Clearinghouse)
http://www.aacap.org	American Academy of Child and Adolescent Psychiatry, Practice parameters
http://www.thecochranelibrary.com	The Cochrane Library

Other medicine resources

www.nelm.nhs.uk	The National electronic library for medicines

www.ukmi.nhs.uk	The UK medicines information network website
www.bnf.org.uk	The British National formula (available as an app)
http://www.toxbase.org	UK National Poisons Information Service

Useful reference books in psychiatry

Taylor D, Paton C, Kapur S. The Maudsley Prescribing guidelines 11th edition
Chichester: Wiley-Blackwell: 2012. (e-book available)

Bazire S. Psychotropic Drug Directory 2013/14
Stratford-upon-Avon: Lloyd-Reinhold Communications LLP: 2013

Stahl S. Stahl's Essential Psychopharmacology: Neuroscientific Basis and Practical Applications
Cambridge: Cambridge University Press 2013

Cowen P, Harrison P, Burns T. Shorter Oxford Textbook of Psychiatry
Oxford: OUP Oxford: 2012

Other medicines related textbooks

Baxter K. Stockley's Drug Interactions 9th edition
London : Pharmaceutical Press: 2010

Briggs G, Freeman R, Yaffe S. Drugs in Pregnancy and Lactation. 9th revised edition
Philadelphia: Lippincott Williams and Wilkins: 2011

Psychiatric journals' home pages

http://archpsyc.jamanetwork.com	JAMA Psychiatry (formerly The Archives of General Psychiatry)
http://ajp.psychiatryonline.org	The American Journal of Psychiatry
http://bjp.rcpsych.org	The British Journal of Psychiatry
http://publications.cpa-apc.org	The Canadian Journal of Psychiatry
http://www.psychiatrist.com	The Clinical Journal of Psychiatry
http://pb.rcpsych.org	The Psychiatrist

Publisher homepages (for many other psychiatric journals)

http://onlinelibrary.wiley.com	The Wiley online library (Acta Psychiatrica Scandinavica)
http://www.sagepub.com	Sage Publications (The Journal of Psychopharmacology, Therapeutic Advances in Psychopharmacology)
http://www.oxfordjournals.org	Oxford Journals (Schizophrenia Bulletin)
http://www.elsevier.com	Elsevier (Biological Psychiatry, The Journal of Affective Disorders, Schizophrenia Research)
http://www.sciencedirect.com	Science direct (European Psychiatry, European Neuropsychopharmacology)
http://adisonline.com	Adis online (CNS Drugs)
https://www.thieme-connect.com	Thieme (Pharmacopsychiatry)
http://journals.lww.com	Lippincott, Williams and Wilkins (The Journal of Clinical Psychopharmacology, International Clinical Psychopharmacology)

Index

M

N

O

P

Q

R

S